$\dfrac{8}{78}$ £8-70

George H. Shames / Donald B. Egolf
UNIVERSITY OF PITTSBURGH

OPERANT CONDITIONING AND THE MANAGEMENT OF STUTTERING

A Book for Clinicians

Prentice-Hall, Inc., *Englewood Cliffs, New Jersey*

Library of Congress Cataloging in Publication Data

SHAMES, GEORGE H. (date)
 Operant conditioning and the management of stuttering.

  Bibliography: p. 173.
  Includes index.
  1. Stuttering. 2. Speech therapy. I. Egolf,
Donald B. (date) joint author. II. Title.
[DNLM: 1. Conditioning, Operant. 2. Stuttering—
Therapy. WM475 S5280]
RC424.S555   616.8′554   75-14346
ISBN 0-13-637322-4

10 9 8 7 6 5 4 3 2 1

Printed in the United States of America

Prentice-Hall International, Inc., *London*
Prentice-Hall of Australia, Pty. Ltd., *Sydney*
Prentice-Hall of Canada, Ltd., *Toronto*
Prentice-Hall of India Private Limited, *New Delhi*
Prentice-Hall of Japan, Inc., *Tokyo*
Prentice-Hall of Southeast Asia (Pte.) Ltd., *Singapore*

Contents

PART III   NEW DIRECTIONS AND CONSIDERATIONS

Preface

Our concern in this book is the improvement of management techniques for the problem of stuttering. An important part of this concern is our hope that this book will encourage meaningful dialogue between clinicians and researchers. If the clinical problems associated with stuttering are to be resolved, the wisdom of both groups will be required.

In the attempt to improve clinical procedures, our activities follow a path quite similar to that of scientific activity in general: we observe stutterers and the available information on stuttering; we think of ideas or hypotheses relating to treatment; we test these ideas or hypotheses; and, on the basis of our test results, we sort through the therapeutic strategies, tagging those that are successful and those that are not. The process is a cyclical one. However, with each revolution or with each pass through the path of observation, idea formulation, idea testing, and idea confirmation, we hope to be closer to resolution or at least closer to having established efficacious therapeutic procedures.

In addition to being guided by the principles associated with scientific thinking, we are further directed in our activities by behavioristic principles, particularly those principles falling under the category of operant conditioning. The term *operant conditioning* creates in many people a vision of some Orwellian world where all behavior is monitored and controlled. This fearful vision is, we believe, unwarranted. First of all, people who are actually involved in applying conditioning procedures to human behavior are many times surprised at the extent to which other people believe in the conditioner's power.

It is usually overestimated. Second, we are concerned only with the person who seeks help. Thus, our goal in using operant conditioning principles is to help an individual go from the backwaters and eddies into the mainstream of life. If we exercise control at all, it is to give the individual seeking help control in return. Albert Schweitzer said in *Reverence for Life* (New York: Philosophical Library, 1965) :

> A man must not try to force his way into the personality of another. To analyse others—unless it be to help back to a sound mind someone who is in spiritual or intellectual confusion—is a rude commencement, for there is a modesty of the soul which we must recognize, just as we do that of the body (pp. 6–7) .

We agree with Schweitzer, and while our mission is not one of spiritual restoration, it is restoration nonetheless. We intrude, therefore, only to restore.

The book is divided into three parts. Part I deals with the principles of operant conditioning and the issues surrounding their application to the clinical problem of stuttering. It is in this part that we hope the value of a researcher-clinician dialogue will emerge. Part II is composed of clinical applications, both group and individual. Here we reveal our clinical attempts in the hopes that clinicians can fuse their clinical experiences with ours. Ideally this fusion will produce a new perception of the clinical process. In Part III we look at what others are doing, what new possibilities are emerging, and from this panoramic view, suggest strategies that we might try, to further refine and improve therapeutic procedures. We believe that information, perhaps like uranium, has a half-life. Data, most particularly, have the shortest half-life. Therefore, of the three parts of this book, we anticipate that Part II will be the most short-lived. Data quickly vanish as subsequent clinical experiments build on past findings and yield better clinical outcomes. Theories and principles have much longer life spans, and like volcanoes, may even lie dormant for many years before they erupt again. Therefore, when a particular therapeutic strategy is unsuccessful, it is most often the strategy that is sacrificed and not the theory from which it was derived.

We are indebted to many individuals as we present this book. There are those who by their writings have taught us. Included here are the many workers, theorists, and researchers in the field of stuttering and in the field of psychology. They are obviously too numerous to list here, but the citations in the text testify to their contributions. We received immeasurable assistance from Janet Blind, Dr. Joseph Carrier, Dr. Peter Johnson, Arlene Kasprisin, Dr. Robert Rhodes, and Dr. Bruce Ryan, all of whom worked with us as graduate students, and from Yvonne Shutak, who served as our research assistant. We also express appreciation to Sondra Chester for her assistance in preparing this manuscript, Barbara Hess, our typist, and Father James L. Aaron and the Catholic Diocese of Pittsburgh for making facilities available for conducting some of the research. Finally, we wish to acknowledge the support given to conduct the research herein described. Grantors were the United States Office of Education (Project No. 482130) and Social and Rehabilitation Services, Department of Health, Education and Welfare (Project No. RD-2274-S) .

I

GENERAL
PRINCIPLES
AND
ISSUES

1

Introduction
to Part I

THE CHALLENGE

Communication behavior in general, and the problem of stuttering in particular, must be viewed within the context of social interactions and interpersonal relationships. When therapy is structured so that interviews are the primary vehicle for interaction, then the give and take of conversational speech between a stutterer and a clinician becomes such a social and interpersonal experience. The primary purpose of this book is to provide for speech clinicians a view of therapy for stuttering through the principles of operant behavior and the techniques of operant conditioning as applied to an interview structure of therapy. Conditioning within such social and interpersonal relationships is far from a simple and discrete stimulus-response, trial 1, trial 2 arrangement. Rather, it is quite complicated and as difficult to achieve as it is to analyze. But it is within these social processes of therapy and the associated conversational contexts of stuttering that we have approached our task. Stuttering, after all, is a problem that exists in a social, conversational, speaking environment, and its modification during therapy must take cognizance of this fact.

It might be well from the start to distinguish between (1) that which has come to be known as operant conditioning, and (2) the clinical application of the principles which underlie operant conditioning.

Operant conditioning refers to a rather well defined set of experimental operations for providing contingencies in order to control and predict behavior. Specifically, it refers to a process of reinforcement whereby the frequency of a particular class of behaviors can be increased or decreased or maintained at a designated level by presenting or withdrawing certain stimuli immediately after a designated response has been emitted. The consequent stimulus (which follows the designated response) is presented only when a previously designated response is emitted and its presentation is, therefore, contingent on the emission of that response. When predicted changes in frequency of responses are observed in association with a schedule of presentation of contingent stimuli or events, we might then infer that operant conditioning has taken place. This is a highly controlled experimental procedure in which evoking stimuli, situational stimuli, response topography, contingent stimuli, the subject's history, and the experimenter's behavior are described, controlled, and/or varied as systematically and as precisely as possible.

On the other hand, the clinical application of the principles which underlie operant conditioning, because of its therapeutic context, may necessarily be less controlled and even violate some of the desired experimental arrangements. In therapy, the previous history of a stutterer cannot be controlled in the way that the history of a laboratory animal can be controlled. Also, the fact that we share a language with the stutterer and that he talks to us and we listen during therapy may, in fact, interfere with our being able to attend to certain designated responses. Such distractions, of course, do not occur in working with animals. Moreover, it appears that much of what takes place in an interview resists being scheduled and is, perhaps, more under the control of the stutterer than of the clinician. These are important distinctions and therefore result in different expectations in the therapy room and in the laboratory. Pointing out these distinctions and expectations might ease the feelings of purists, who believe that the term operant conditioning should be restricted for use only in the highly controlled laboratory operation where human judgment and human error are minimized by the use of timers, counters, relays, switches, and cumulative recorders. An awareness of the differences between the laboratory and the clinic might also encourage the clinician who does not want to be stringently programmed, does not wish to become a slave to a schedule of activity, and does not wish to give up his most prized possession, his freedom to hypothesize and to formulate and act on judgments made during clinical sessions. In short, the clinician should not try to replicate the laboratory. This book is not designed to create a new breed of operant conditioners, but rather to help clinicians learn a set of behavioral principles and some of the tactics and techniques of operant conditioning that may be selectively applied to clinical problems.

There is a challenge here, however, for both the clinician and the experimentalist. The clinician's claims that research is too remote from the real world of life's stresses, and that too often research data never find their way to any clinical application, are all too familiar. These, perhaps, are justifiable claims, which for the most part, appear to be directed at the content or substantive information of research findings. In the instance of the operant model, we find that the experimentalist and the clinician are moving closer and closer together, not merely because of the content of research findings, but because the tactics, the strategies, and the specific operations of the researcher appear to be directly relevant to the tactics, the strategies, and the specific operations of the clinician. Even a cursory consideration shows obvious similarities between the clinician and the operant researcher. Both attempt to assess the representativeness of their observations. Both introduce into their situations and analyze the effects of independent variables upon speech. Both analyze the occasions for particular speech responses to determine what variables might control those responses. Both attempt to shape behavior toward some desired end, and both observe relations between the speaker, his speech responses, and the consequent reactions of listeners. The challenge is to discover whether the clinician can advantageously utilize the tactics of the experimentalist. As this convergence develops, let us not be afraid of collisions, or afraid of mistakes. They will most certainly occur, but they can easily be converted into productive interactions of greater relevance for the researcher and more efficient tactics for the clinician. It is the tactics of operant conditioning that may be relevant and the principles underlying these tactics that may have clinical value in the hands of speech clinicians, not necessarily the particular forms that these tactics have taken in the research laboratory.

We plan to embed our considerations of these techniques and principles of conditioning within clinical material and clinical processes. At the same time, however, we want you to recognize the operant bases of our discussions and the many diverse possibilities for application of these principles to therapy. Such recognition is neither whimsical nor arbitrary, but rather could make the difference between your becoming an imitator of the techniques described, or an applier of principles of behavior and, therefore, an innovator of therapeutic techniques.

A GLIMPSE OF OUR RECORD

Any serious consideration of the problem of stuttering necessarily involves a sensitivity to its long history and persistence over many generations. Stuttering has revealed an endurance historically and individually that has proven frustrating to the stutterer, to the clinician, to the theorist, and to the researcher. Pessimism and doubt would be reasonable reactions to such a history. However, these reactions to the past are at the same time tempered by what we have learned from our past experiences with therapy for stuttering, by the most recent advances in knowledge and information about people, and how and why people behave the way they do. We have a distinct advantage of having the observations, theory, and information of our predecessors to help us. Let us briefly examine the record and review some of the clinical and personal experiences we at one time or another may have shared.

We have been exposed to, although we may not have learned and adopted, several frames of reference and languages for observing and characterizing the problem of stuttering. We are referring, specifically, to the many theories of the nature of stuttering. To name just a few, we have the semantic theory (Johnson, 1958); the approach-avoidance conflict theory (Sheehan, 1958b); the psychoanalytic theory (Blanton, 1958; Coriat, 1958); the visual imagery theory (Swift, 1958); the negative emotionality theory (Brutten and Shoemaker, 1967); and the organic and constitutional theories (Van Riper, 1958; West, 1958; Boome, 1958; Bryngelson, 1958; Greene, 1958). Many of these theories have proven extremely valuable. These frames of reference have sorted out and focused on a number of events, both overt and covert, that have proven to be significant aspects and dimensions of stuttering. They have helped us to organize our thinking about the problem, and as a result, have been related to the successes of some clinicians. On the other hand, we have acquired so many languages and dimensions to characterize stuttering that each frame of reference begins to interfere with the others, insofar as understanding the problem and applying these ideas to therapy are concerned.

Our theories of the problem and our procedures in clinical management often form nebulous aggregates with very little relationship to one another. We have the theory in one compartment, and our therapeutic procedures in another compartment. At times, there appears to be very little relationship between what one might expect to be the therapeutic and clinical outgrowth of the theory we espouse, and our actual clinical transactions. For example, it becomes reasonable to ask how the "bounce technique" of therapy relates to the semantic theory of stuttering; or how alleged therapeutic comments like "accept yourself as a stutterer" can be reconciled with an anxiety-reduction reinforcement theory of therapy; or how clinicians can move from "instructional activity" during therapy to client-centered counseling activity with the same stutterer. These illustrative pairings of seemingly opposing concepts and tactics are a part of our clinical history and can still be frequently observed in current therapeutic practices.

Our successes and failures with individual stutterers have been only occasionally clearly understood. At times, the outcome of therapy was attributed to some kind of reality testing or to situational desensitization, with very little concern or regard about how these clinical tactics fit into a theoretical model. At other times, it appeared that the outcome of therapy was due to a series of almost ritualistic and superstitiously based phonetic and motor exercises. At still other times, the manipulation of the young stutterer's home environment was thought crucial. Of course, there was always the chance that the stutterer had learned to talk about himself and about his speech differently, either through some directive confrontation with an advising clinician, or through some directive process of client-centered counseling. Then there is always the variable of individual clinical style, and for want of a better term, the therapist's personality, which may have been the overriding influence. And there is always luck, divine providence, and the drive of the stutterer to help himself. In short, we have not separated the technique from the principles underlying the technique, from the dispenser of the technique. With such a state of affairs, replication of clinical procedures is difficult but still necessary if we are to understand our work and improve our effectiveness.

Probably the most profound aspects of the record, however, were the results of therapy. Hard data about therapeutic outcomes are difficult to come by for a number of reasons. There have been technical problems of measurement and assessment, lack of agreement about what constitutes therapeutic progress, lack of interest in follow-up studies, difficulties in obtaining representative samples of subjects, and so on. Thus, we continue to find ourselves relying on nonrepresentative anecdotal accounts, some of which report good results while others report poor results.

The time is long overdue for describing and assessing this process we have been calling therapy for stuttering. This does not necessarily mean that we discard our current therapeutic procedures, but rather that we learn from them, add to them, and modify them.

DECISIONS FACING THE CLINICIAN

A discussion of decision-making can sink quickly to the bedrock issues of free will and determinism. Briefly, the classical controversy between free will and determinism can be stated in terms of man's ability to make choices governing his conduct and behavior or lack of ability to do so. Those espousing the free-will view believe that man can chart his own destiny while determinists believe that man is helplessly skidding along through life at the mercy of external forces, be they physical, psychological, or suprahuman.

While it is not our purpose to pursue a discussion of the free-will versus determinism controversy here, stimulating though it may be, we do find some elements here to have operational value. In doing so we will accept E. G. Boring's dictum that freedom is equivalent to ignorance (Boring, 1957) :

> . . . freedom, when you believe it is operating, always resides in an area of ignorance. If there is a known law, you do not have freedom. . . . (p. 190)

At first reading, this rather cryptic comment may seem a jarring juxtaposition of words like "good murderer." Freedom which we cherish is equated with ignorance which we abhor.

However, if a patient were affected with an infection that was readily treatable with a nonreactive antibiotic and if a physician failed to use the available treatment, the physician would be suspect, would be regarded as ignorant. In like manner, if there were a cure for stuttering and if we as clinicians failed to administer the treatment associated with this cure, we would be regarded as unprofessional. We may plead in our defense that we were exercising our free will. In doing so, however, we would be behaving, in Boring's sense, ignorantly, because we failed to utilize the available information.

Even a cursory survey of the literature on stuttering reveals a sea of ignorance. For example, a clinician can choose from a countless number of theories on causality, maintenance, remediation, and relapse. This freedom to choose is a manifestation of our ignorance on the topic. It is the purpose of this section to examine the clinician's decision-making behavior in line with the preceding comments. Specifically, how does a clinician use available information about himself, his clients, and about stuttering in general in arriving at decisions?

The person who enters the profession of speech pathology has made a series of decisions before meeting his first stutterer. Perhaps the most important of these was the decision to embark upon a professional career. Although for many of us this decision was made in the past, it still can have present implications. For example, a decision to enter the profession might have been based on a personal experience with the problem of stuttering or some other communication disorder. Perhaps a member of the immediate family or a friend stuttered and we witnessed the shame and suffering attendant with the disorder. We wanted to do something, and a large part of this "doing something" was entering the profession. A second possibility might be that we touched upon the field only tangentially and became interested. For instance, we might have used stutterers as subjects in a psychological study and became so interested we decided to work with them clinically and professionally. A third kind of decision is perhaps the more common. Included here are practical "bread and butter" type decisions. Scholarships were available in the field, vacancies were open, or the field of speech pathology seemed generally attractive.

The reasons underlying the decision to enter the field probably have implications for subsequent decision-making behavior. For example, in choosing training institutions, some will choose those with a strong research orientation; others will seek those staffed by former stutterers; while still others will gravitate to those institutions where there are vacancies and/or scholarship opportunities.

As one proceeds from deciding upon a profession to deciding upon a training institution to actual training and practice, it is possible that biases can accrue. By bias accretion is meant the systematic rejection of valid information. This rejection may be deliberate or unwitting. In most cases it is the latter.

At this point in the discussion the clinician may feel that he is ignorant, in that there is no single efficacious method for the treatment of stuttering, so necessarily his decisions must be based on personal preferences, beliefs, and attitudes, as well as practical matters. In short, how can we justifiably ask the clinician to make the correct decision when the field of speech pathology is ignorant (again in Boring's sense). The information for making the single correct decision is just not available.

The resolution to this dilemma seems to be that clinicians must first be flexible enough to question what they are presently doing; must second seek the best information available; and must third apply in a systematic way forthcoming new knowledge. To be flexible, to be able to question one's behavior, means that one is willing to shed one's biases, and have one's behavior determined by the best available information.

There are still difficulties, however, even if we shed our biases. The difficulty lies with the term best available information. In an area where there are contradictory but equally plausible ideas, it is difficult to evaluate information; it is time-consuming, and difficult on methodological grounds, particularly in the therapeutic arena, where longitudinal studies may be required.

A more complex and complicating factor deals with the aura or enthusiasm that accompanies the publication of any new information such as new therapeutic procedures. Some philosophers would say that we can never distinguish between what is true and what we have been persuaded to believe is true. Bloodstein (1969) has stated this problem:

> The fact that the stutterer may be helped for some time by practically any type of therapy in which he believes strongly has some implications that

should be carefully noted. It means that he may be especially likely to obtain short-term benefit from a therapist who is deeply convinced of the effectiveness of his methods, who happens to be endowed with charisma, or who has a prestigious role (e.g., physician, psychiatrist, or the like). A corollary hypothesis for which there appears to be more than a little evidence in the history of treatment of stuttering is that almost every new movement in therapy is likely to enjoy a kind of honeymoon during which successes occur in part as a result of the hope and enthusiasms of clinicians. To the extent that this is true, evaluating the results of any new departure in therapy is obviously no simple matter. (p. 240)

In spite of all the aforementioned problems of assessing the validity of new or available information, the clinician must continue to make this assessment. And as previously suggested, the first step in performing this assessment is to question one's current professional behavior. Of course the ideal state of affairs would be to be free of ignorance. In such a state there would be no need for assessment. One could imagine in this state the existence of a single therapy program that would be universally effective in the elimination of stuttering. We are, obviously, far from the ideal. However, in the construction of therapy programs we approach this ideal. The comprehensive therapy program is decision-free, and when in operation the decision branches have been preplanned or programmed. In programmed therapy the clinician does not ask what he should do today but, on the basis of the stutterer's last performance, what does the program dictate that he do today. When constructing therapy programs we bring a new systematization to the process. Since our steps and strategies must be preplanned, we are forced to make a pretherapy comprehensive analysis of the decisions we will encounter during therapy. Programming has revealed to many clinicians the decisions they have actually made in therapy, some apparently without awareness.

CRITERIA FOR SELECTING AND EVALUATING A THERAPY FOR STUTTERING

How do we detach ourselves and look at something we have been doing for several years with a view toward changing and improving? How do we select from the numerous possibilities available to us in the literature? The most obvious first step is to evolve some criteria for evaluating the attributes and merits of a particular therapy. Certain questions must be asked about therapy that tell us whether it is valid and reliable. In order to understand and effectively apply therapy, we must know what is being fed into the system by the stutterer, by us as clinicians, and by the ideas we hold about the problem. We are suggesting that we ask ourselves a series of questions that may serve as criteria to help us decide upon the value and usefulness of a particular therapy.

QUESTION 1:
IS THE THERAPY RELATED
TO A THEORETICAL POINT OF VIEW?

Implicit in this question is the need to adopt *some* point of view about the nature of stuttering that is correlated and integrated within an operational orientation about the therapy process. Although there are many diverse points of view about stuttering, and although some of us operate more comfortably with one rather than another, the mere fact of diversity does not invalidate any point of view. What really is the importance of having a point of view? We could, after all, operate as technique hunters. A point of view provides us with a way to grasp the substantive content of the problem. Each frame of reference puts us in touch with the pertinent events of stuttering. Each point of view provides a vocabulary and a set of rules for characterizing stuttering, and for characterizing people. It directs us to the things we look for and find. It focuses our attention on things that we might otherwise not perceive at all. It should provide long-term strategies and goals for the individual stutterer as he operates in our rather complex society, as well as provide short-term operational tactics for use during therapy sessions. For a frame of reference to be functional, it should generate hypotheses about relations among our perceptions which we can then test during therapy and with which we can, hopefully, benefit the stutterer. In this sense, a frame of reference about stuttering is the central organizing core or nucleus of ideas around which therapy is built. Without a theoretical point of view about the nature of stuttering, our clinical activities become nothing more than inconsistent and ultimately ineffective trial-and-error rituals. Sometimes, of course, we may find that serendipitously a particular technique for a particular stutterer may be quite beneficial. However, when a clinical technique is not successful, and when that technique is not derived from a theory, it is very difficult to analyze the failure. When a technique is part of a set of underlying principles, we can go back to those principles to modify the technique or the direction of our activities appropriately.

Our theory should lead us to a set of clinical strategies by defining the dynamics of the stuttering problem. For example, if our theory states that stuttering involves some relations between anticipatory phenomena

(Bloodstein, 1958) and overt speech behavior, then our observations, our interpretations, and our clinical activity should focus dead center on *these* events and relations. On the other hand, if we feel that stuttering is maintained because it benefits the stutterer (Rubin and Culatta, 1971; Shames and Sherrick, 1963) then it is these relations which will occupy our attention during therapy.

It is not our purpose to catalog the many hypotheses that have been offered about factors that relate to and control stuttering. As we know, they range from the various psychoanalytic views of stutterers as neurotics (Travis, 1957; Krout, 1936; Coriat, 1958; Glauber, 1958), through learning theory conceptualizations that view stuttering as operant behavior (Flanagan, Goldiamond, and Azrin, 1959; Shames and Sherrick, 1963; Siegel, 1970), or as being maintained by anxiety reduction (Wischner, 1950), or as functions of negative emotion (Brutten and Shoemaker, 1967), all the way to theories of physiological predisposition (West, 1958; Van Riper, 1958). Hopefully, the particular theory each of us adopts as the foundation for organizing our clinical work has research data as evidence of its validity. Whichever of these points of view we embrace, each one binds us to a system of thought, to a set of observations and events, to a system of asking questions, and, hopefully, to a system of therapy.

QUESTION 2:
DOES THE THEORETICAL POINT OF VIEW
LEAD TO STRATEGIES FOR THERAPY
AND PROVIDE A DESCRIPTION
OF OPERATIONAL TACTICS?

Now that we have a theoretical handle to the problem of stuttering—now that we see it as avoidance behavior, as anticipatory stress, as approach-avoidance conflict, as disturbed social interaction, as a function of its consequences and effects—now that we have focused on what we feel are the significant dimensions of stuttering, what do we do about them in a therapeutic context? How does information about these things become available to us during therapy, and how do we then deal with that information for the ultimate benefit of the stutterer?

There are numerous ideas available about the process of therapy, that is, the strategies and tactics for changing the stutterer's behavior. It is easy to become overwhelmed by the many ways in which the process of therapy has been characterized and can be dimensionalized. It is one thing to say that we must eliminate avoidance behavior, or change the feelings of a stutterer, or change the home environment; but it is something else to accomplish these goals. How do we change feelings? How do we modify a home environment? How do we eliminate avoidance behavior?

In clinical reports as well as in research, we often hear allusions to such things as dependency, support, individual responsibility, confrontation, punishment, positive reinforcement, acceptance, empathy, transference, resistance, interpretation, directiveness, and client-centeredness. Each of these terms suggests a way of looking at processes that take place during therapy designed to achieve our goals. Unfortunately, very often these terms are not clearly defined operationally or they may involve a kind of mental jump, where inference is built upon inference with little or no description of the reasoning process or behavior involved.

It is quite conceivable that no one process orientation can help all stutterers, but that each stutterer may require his own somewhat unique system. Or it may well be that there are some elements of the process of therapy common to all, but that each stutterer may require some individualized variation. In a sense, we must read each individual stutterer and ask ourselves some questions about the most appropriate way of interacting with him.

Do we nurture and support a particular stutterer in his mode of behaving so that we can gain his trust and confidence, and enable him to examine painful material as we gradually move him along through some aversive self-insights? Do we become the authoritative father figure, and therefore evaluate, react, and confront the stutterer with his behavior or with our own reactions as a listener even though we are his therapist? Do we merely let him talk and when he says something that fits into our scheme of viewing the problem, then respond with some punishing comment like "I don't understand," or a reinforcing comment like "I agree"? Or, do we set the stage for certain kinds of behavior by providing occasions for their occurrence through questions or instructions, and then evaluate the stutterer's performance? Do we see the process as always involving our ability to communicate our interest and concern? Do we see therapy exclusively as an activity of interviewing or do we plan a sequence of encounters whereby talking about stuttering, examining the problem, and changing the way the stutterer characterizes it during interviews, functions as a type of verbal readiness program that must lead to a program of action, outside of the context of the interview, in the social milieu of the stutterer?

These are merely a few illustrations of the sorts of issues we should be dealing with as clinicians and researchers of the clinical process. If we wish to change what is going on, we must be able to characterize the process as a whole and the interaction in particular as a part of the total system, and systematically manipulate those aspects of it that will result in an optimal arrangement.

QUESTION 3:
DOES THE THERAPY RESULT IN A CHANGE
IN STUTTERING OR THE BEHAVIOR
ASSOCIATED WITH IT?

The answer to this question is directly related to the first two questions, in that it deals with the way we view the problem of stuttering and the task of therapy. We feel that we must keep in mind the fact that we are dealing with a *speech* problem of *stuttering,* which in turn, may give rise to associated behaviors and emotional states (avoidance, guilt). Our efforts should be directed toward dealing with *stuttering behavior,* toward those behaviors and emotional states associated with stuttering, and toward those factors that appear to exercise some control over its development and continuance. Many diverse problems may be presented to us by stutterers. If we can be of help for those other problems, so much the better. However, if the alleviation of those problems does not result in changes in stuttering and its associated behavior, it is difficult to characterize our ministrations as therapy for stuttering. We should not delude ourselves into thinking that turning out a "happy stutterer" necessarily means that we have engaged in therapy for stuttering. The ultimate question to be answered is whether stuttering behavior and those behaviors and emotional states associated with it are reduced or changed by this therapy.

QUESTION 4:
CAN THE THERAPY BE EVALUATED?

Just as stutterers are not immune to a variety of human problems, clinicians, vulnerable to their own strong needs to help, are also not immune. Although it may seem paradoxical, it becomes easy for a clinician to lose touch with what is going on in therapy. Unless, from the very beginning, some objective system of prompt feedback to the clinician is established to tell us about the stutterer's progress, as well as about the interaction process, we may find ourselves intensively involved in irrelevance. We must stay in touch with what is happening in therapy if we want to provide the most effective therapeutic experience. Most of the time, our general awareness of what is happening results in anecdotal memories and reports. Although these evaluative impressions may be valuable as a general guide and starting place, they should be made more precise, since our need to see the stutterer as improving can so easily color them. It is not enough to say that the stutterer is improving, or not improving, and leave it at that. How is he showing this improvement or lack of it? How can we document our observations? What is the evidence? We might go on to say that he is stuttering less or in a different way. We might even become so bold as to define what the term "less stuttering" means in terms of frequency, and describe the numerous circumstances under which these frequencies were observed, both before, during, and after therapy. We might characterize in a descriptive as well as a quantitative way the stutterer's social behavior, his avoidance behavior, or the language he uses to talk about himself and his world. Very often we might find that our general impressions are not in agreement with more descriptive or quantitative analyses of therapy and that we are indeed out of touch with what is happening.

QUESTION 5:
CAN THE THERAPY BE REVISED
AND ACTIVITIES MODIFIED
IN A SYSTEMATIC AND ORDERLY FASHION?

There are times when our feedback system will tell us that the stutterer is not making progress. Given that we have accurately and descriptively assessed the status of the stutterer's behavior, how do we now bring about the desired changes that we have thus far not observed? One way is to recognize, acknowledge, or hypothesize, depending on how strongly we feel about what we are doing, that as clinicians we are active participants in the therapeutic process. From the beginning of therapy, we can exercise a great deal of control over the stutterer's behavior, which we manipulate in one way or another by virtue of our presence, to his benefit or to his detriment.

We must grow sensitive to what we do in therapy, to whether we are consistent in what we do and whether our own behavior is related to our observations of what the stutterer does.

QUESTION 6:
DOES THE THERAPY ACCOUNT
FOR THE SOCIAL AND EMOTIONAL CONTEXT
OF THE PROBLEM?

Stuttering neither develops nor exists in a vacuum. Stuttering is a behavioral response of a living, feeling, reacting individual who is operating in some form of socially interactive system with other people. Therapy does not cut out or separate a person's response of stuttering from his functioning in his social system. Although the stutterer's fluency may be changed in the therapy sessions, we must recognize that the therapy room is only one aspect of the stutterer's real world.

Our concerns should include those factors that appear to evoke stuttering as well as those factors that appear to strengthen and maintain stuttering outside the clinic. This is not a problem merely of dealing with the speaker and the way he talks, but also of dealing with the people and events that affect the stutterer. As Wendell Johnson stated (Johnson, 1964), we should try to identify "the members of the problem": the listeners, the reactors, the evaluators, the consequators (those people who provide consequences for stuttering, including the stutterer himself), and when appropriate, to bring them into the therapeutic process.

Finally, we come to the moment of truth of our work and to an answer to the question of whether there is any validity to what we and the stutterers have been engrossed in, that is, a consideration of what is happening outside the clinic room in the real social and talking life of the stutterer.

We know that it is quite common to observe changes in behavior that are specific to certain situational circumstances. We know that stutterers may speak and behave one way with us, his clinicians, and another way with his family, friends, and employer.

Some clinicians feel that it is the sole responsibility of the stutterer to carry over into the real world the changes he has made in the clinic room with the clinician. Others feel quite the opposite, that this phase of dealing with stuttering requires as much, although possibly different, participation by the clinician. Whichever your disposition might be, however, there are questions of clinical strategy to be considered. Do we work in a type of laboratory situation which is artificial and remote from the real life social stresses that we all face? Do we remain in this context until the stutterer reaches some final form of behavior as though we were preparing him for a debut at a coming-out party? Do we keep an eye on the possibilities of social carryover at every step so that the boundaries for the stutterer's behavior are not restrained by artificially and clinically imposed barriers from the start?

This situational approach, of course, requires much planning and is more complicated than the interaction that takes place in the therapy room. One of the most difficult aspects of dealing with this issue is the initial evaluation of the stutterer's behavior in social and emotional situations. Real situational measurement, that is, measurements in the real-life situations of the stutterer, of even the frequency of stuttering, is most difficult to arrange. The systematic observation of the stutterer's social behavior in terms other than often imprecise introspective reports or written answers to paper and pencil tests are also extremely difficult to come by. And yet, such assessments before, during, and after therapy are necessary if we wish to determine the effects of our efforts to facilitate or systematically program situational carryover. This apart from philosophical reservations is a social engineering problem and a problem of social measurement that we believe can eventually be resolved once its importance is acknowledged.

Given the resolution of this measurement problem, there is the strategy of carryover. In many cases, carryover procedures seem like afterthoughts, either in the form of clinicians' suggestions for the stutterer to be carried out independently or some ad hoc activities to be carried out under the clinician's supervision. We believe that carryover is a part of therapy involving both the stutterer and the clinician. The process revolves around the original conceptions and relations we hypothesize about the nature of stuttering and about the process of therapy. The clinician may justifiably see and implement his role in situational carry-over right from the start as that of gradually weaning the stutterer from a highly controlled, nonthreatening situation in the clinic, through situations that are more complicated, less controlled, and initially, more threatening. This weaning sequence may repeat itself over and over again, until the situations at home, at work, on the street, or in the therapy room are viewed by the stutterer as communicatively similar. The clinician gradually withdraws his support, thus facilitating the emergence of independent behavior on the part of the stutterer.

SUMMARY

We have formulated six basic questions that might be asked about any therapy for stuttering. The answers to these questions could well serve as criteria for judging the usefulness of a therapy. It follows that we should be asking and answering the very same questions about the therapy described in this book. Following our presentation of the operant approach and illustrative case studies derived from it, we shall similarly scrutinize our own approach in terms of these criteria.

2

Operant Conditioning and the Clinical Problem of Stuttering

STUTTERING AS OPERANT BEHAVIOR

Operant conditioning is not a term that has just appeared on the horizon, but it may be new to many of us in the field of speech therapy. The probable reason for this is that, as clinicians, we have been more concerned with human behavior and human problems than we have with animal behavior and the numerous problems that researchers have created for rats and pigeons. Gradually, however, the principles of operant behavior have been applied in trying to understand how people learn and acquire certain types of behavior. These developments, of course, have become too tempting for some of us to ignore, and research on human learning through operant conditioning has expanded so that it now includes research on the *problems* we have in being human.

The therapies described in this book are based on the ideas that the development and maintenance, and the therapy, of stuttering can be profitably viewed within the framework of the principles of operant conditioning (Shames and Sherrick, 1963). Although this may resemble a theory of stuttering, it is erroneous to think of these ideas as a theoretical position about stuttering. As a procedure for categorizing behavior, operant analysis may resemble the procedures of any theory of stuttering by which events are placed in relation to one another. However, there appear to be at least two basic differences between the application of traditional theories of stuttering and the application of operant principles to this problem. One of these is that an operant analysis requires a minimal number of assumptions and inferences regarding the events that are observed and the principles underlying these events.

A second important difference is that this frame of reference offers no content information about which events should be observed and classified, and eventually, manipulated. Operant conditioning principles may tell us *how* to manipulate, but not *what* to manipulate. The form and content of operant transactions and strategies do not come from principles of manipulation. Viewing stuttering as operant behavior does not deny those observable events significant to content theories of stuttering. In fact, an operant analysis depends on these events for its basic character. The specific forms of responses, the occasions for responses and the forms of the consequential events following stuttering depend first of all on the obervations of those people who are immersed in the problem; namely the stutterer, his community of listeners, and the speech clinicians who have been attempting to manage this behavior.

By reexamining a number of the events encountered in the clinical problem of stuttering and casting them into operant conditioning paradigms, we are able to generate a number of testable hypotheses and experiments concerning the relations among these events, the results of which may ultimately be applied to clinical management.

If we take a closer look at those events encountered in the problem of stuttering, we see that they can be roughly grouped into several categories. Of paramount importance, and certainly those events which have occupied most of our attention, are those that characterize the speaker, that is, the stutterer. We have tried to describe his overt speech behavior, in terms of his rate of speaking, as well as such properties of his speech as repetitions, prolongations, fragmenting of words, forcing, and muscular tension. There has been little agreement that any one of these observable characteristics alone constitutes what people call stuttering. There have also been attempts to characterize a number of private events, which are not usually made public or observable. These have included selection and rejection of words and attitudes, fear, anxiety, anticipation, and rehearsal. These events, because they are not directly observed, are sometimes inferred as taking place on the basis of either a theoretical assumption, or on the basis of an interpretation of something that has been observed.

A second category of information encountered in the problem of stuttering deals with the circumstances during which stuttering responses are emitted. In this sphere, attention has been given to such antecedent events as the specific words, speaking situations, emotional states, and people that appear to be the occasions for stuttering responses and seem to evoke them.

Still a third category of clinical attention involves the behavior of the listener. There has been concern over the listener's evaluation of the speech of young children and how this evaluation may influence that speech behavior. There has also been concern over the stutterer as his own listener and self-evaluator, and how this feedback influences his speech. These consequent events of stuttering have been known to speech clinicians for some time and attempts have been made to manipulate them in therapy as a technique for modifying the speech behavior of stutterers. With young children these therapeutic activities have been directed toward manipulating the consequent behavior of parents, teachers, and siblings with relatively effective results. With adults who stutter, therapeutic attention has concentrated on manipulating the stutterer as his own listener and evaluator with a great deal less success.

What we have briefly tried to do here, by mentioning only a few of the content variables encountered in the clinical problem of stuttering, is illustrate how these traditional clinical observations fall into categories that resemble the category system of operant analysis (i.e., antecedent events → stuttering responses → consequent events) and lead us quite easily into viewing stuttering in this way. The significant difference between these clinical observations and the operant system is that in the operant system, contingency relations can be hypothesized and studied in a systematic way among these three categories of events.

The principles of operant conditioning and the techniques of behavior modification have been applied to the problem of stuttering in a number of ways. In fact, there are so many profoundly different ways in which operant conditioning has been applied to stuttering, we might justifiably think that these attempts are unrelated to one another and have very little, if anything, in common. This is not the case. There is a commonality among these different operant endeavors. But this commonality appears to be at the level of basic principles, and not necessarily at the level of their clinical or research application.

Underlying all of the operant enterprises is the basic idea that on certain occasions the frequency of certain kinds of behavior is influenced by the consequences generated by that behavior. This basic behavioral theme relates behavior to the events that immediately precede and immediately follow it.

The manner in which operant procedures are applied to the problem of stuttering can and has covered a broad range of events. Each operant approach may have different goals, may focus on different aspects of stuttering behavior, and may arrange different ingenious ways for modifying that behavior. It might, therefore, be a serious mistake to lump all operant approaches under one umbrella, even though they share a shelter of underlying principles.

THE TERMS
OF OPERANT CONDITIONING

The principles of operant behavior do not constitute a theory of stuttering, but rather a set of principles about behavior in general. Very simply, operant behavior is that behavior whose frequency or probability of occurrence is influenced by the consequences it generates. If the behavior is not influenced by its consequences, then it is either not operant behavior, or we have not as yet found the right way to modify it.

The field of operant conditioning has generated a series of terms for characterizing the above processes. As we familiarize ourselves with these terms, we may find that much of the behavior associated with them is already known to us. We come to realize that operant strategies really introduce no new content to our work, but rather dispose us toward more precise observation and definition, toward greater consistency in our behavior as clinicians, and toward developing more objective ways of evaluating the processes and results of therapy.

THE STUTTERER'S RESPONSES
DURING THERAPY INTERVIEWS

Let us first talk about some of those things that are obviously familiar to us: the things that we have observed stutterers do during clinical sessions. Some of these relate to the way the stutterer talks or what he does while talking. At times, he may be relatively fluent, just as we all are. At other times, he may repeat what he says in various ways; he may repeat a syllable or a sound, or an entire word, or several words, or a phrase. He may also prolong certain portions of an utterance or interject an unnecessary sound or group of words that do not contribute to the grammatical integrity of his message. He may be silent for long intervals of time. Some of these behaviors have been termed starters, avoidances, releasers, and postponement devices (Van Riper, 1954). These terms, however, do not describe behavior, but rather interpret the functions of the behavior. For the operant worker, it is the behavioral description and not its functional interpretation that is dealt with, until the function is experimentally verified.

We have also observed things that have come to be known as secondary behavior. These behaviors, when they involve the oral and vocal mechanisms, are very often thought to compete with the relatively fluent flow of speech. They may include what we commonly call struggle behavior, such as excessive muscular tension (pressing the lips together or the tongue against the palate, protruding the tongue, taking a deep breath, locking the vocal cords, constricting the nose, mouth, tongue, or the entire body in various postures of pressure). They may involve other parts of the body, for example, foot stomping, eye blinking, eye squeezing, finger tapping, head shaking, knee slapping, or head turning to avoid eye contact.

Another type of behavior we have observed the stutterer emit relates to what he talks about and how he characterizes his world, that is, the content and themes of his language. We are referring here to his evaluations of himself and his speech, and his attitudes and feelings about his friends, family, and listeners (Williams, 1957; Shames, Egolf, and Rhodes, 1969).

Still another kind of behavior we may have observed the stutterer emit relates to his responses to various kinds of social, speaking, and emotional situations. Some of us perhaps have even observed stutterers at a more basic physiological level (perspiring, EKG, GSR, etc.). In general, we are referring to those observable events that we have agreed to call stuttering or that we think have relevance to the problem.

In looking at the things stutterers do when they speak, or in identifying the responses of stutterers, we consciously or unwittingly categorize different responses into one single functional response category or class. For example, one identified stuttering episode may contain two repetitions of the initial syllable while another may contain five. We usually do not distinguish the former from the latter, but label both episodes as stuttering events belonging to the same response class. The technical term for the response class is an operant. An *operant* is a group or class of responses that we regard as functionally equivalent.

The definition of an operant is important and, although a particular definition may be clear to the experimenter or clinician, the data can offer surprises. If, for instance, we define an operant called stuttering and decide to show disapproval after each occurrence of stuttering, we may observe a decrease in stuttering frequency. However, we may also observe a decrease in verbal output. Thus the actual operant manipulated may not only include stuttering responses but verbal responses in general.

THE CLINICIAN'S RESPONSES
DURING THERAPY INTERVIEWS:
PROVIDING ANTECEDENT
AND CONSEQUENT EVENTS

Therapy usually involves at least two people—the stutterer and the clinician. What are some of the things we as clinicians do during therapeutic interviews? We ask questions. We instruct. We give information. We provide support. We somehow communicate our concern and understanding. We confront. We evaluate. We interpret and provide understandings previously unknown to the stutterer. We reject. We accept, agree, and approve. We prod and prompt for more verbal output. We encourage. We disapprove. We repeat what we have heard, or paraphrase. We speak softly, loudly, or in a questioning style. Sometimes, perhaps not often enough, we remain silent. Such events are very familiar to us.

The point in time and the frequency with which we do these things may have varying effects on the stutterer and the behaviors we associate with the stutterer. The form, timing, and frequency of the clinician's behaviors may determine their therapeutic value. Do these behaviors by a clinician serve as cues or occasions to evoke a particular response by a stutterer? Do these behaviors by the clinician strengthen or weaken desirable and undesirable responses by the stutterer? Or, are some of our responses of little significance to the therapy, but rather a reflection of our own emotional states? Are some of our behaviors in response not to the stutterer, but to our own thinking, with little or no regard for the stutterer's presence?

These are not exhaustive lists of behaviors emitted by the stutterer and by the clinician during therapy. However, the lists are sufficient enough for us to ask about their significance. Does our behavior as a clinician relate in some way to the behavior of the stutterer, and to the changes and growth we want to help to bring about in therapy? This is the crucial question. We propose that we will find some answers to that question through the principles of operant behavior, because these principles require that we experimentally verify the relations between the clinician's behavior in the clinic room and the changes in the stutterer's behavior.

THE OPERANT PARADIGM: INFLUENCING THE STUTTERER'S BEHAVIOR

Let us now look at the operant model and fill in some of the voids by bringing together our clinical behavior and the stutterer's behavior. The simplest way to do this is with a series of diagrams that may characterize the relations between the stutterer's and clinician's behaviors during therapy. In the center of the following diagram, we see an **R**. Let this R stand for the large number of forms that stutterers' behaviors have been observed to take, i.e., the speech, language content, social and emotional, as well as physiologic responses listed above. These speech, language, and social behaviors of the stutterer have histories of development and histories of factors which control their occurrence. Some of

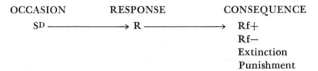

OCCASION   RESPONSE   CONSEQUENCE

S^D ————————→ R ————————→ Rf+

                                Rf−

                                Extinction

                                Punishment

The Paradigms of Operant Conditioning

them may be considered desirable and compatible with the goals of therapy, while others may be considered quite undesirable and possibly incompatible with achieving therapeutic change. The important thing to remember here, is that R stands for an *observable event* that we have agreed to call stuttering behavior, or that we feel is behavior that has relevance to the problem. Most of these are behaviors we may well expect to see the stutterer emit during therapy.

As clinicians, what can we do when we see the stutterer emitting these behaviors? What we do, of course, depends on how we feel about what we see the stutterer do. If we like or approve of his behavior, we can do one thing; if we think that his behavior is undesirable, we can do something else. The clinician's judgments about the desirability of the stutterer's behaviors arise from his theoretical point of view of the problem.

In the diagram, to the right of the R, we see four possible events that could occur after a response and may serve as contingent consequences of a speech (stuttered or fluent) or social response by a stutterer during therapy. These four types of events also represent types of behaviors a clinician might emit in his efforts to modify a stutterer's speech and social behaviors. Basically, the clinician's job is to provide or arrange consequences for the stutterer's speech and social responses. The intended effect of these consequences is to strengthen desirable behavior and to suppress or extinguish undesirable behavior. Very often, for a child who stutters, this may mean intervening in some way with the child's external environment, with his parents, or siblings, or friends, or teachers. For an adult stutterer, however, many of the consequences of speech (stuttered and fluent) may come from the stutterer himself, in the form of cognitive self-evaluations and sensations of tensions. The clinician's job here may well focus on changing consequences, not of the external environment, but those consequences generated within the stutterer in reaction to his own behavior. Or, the clinician, involved with the stutterer during therapy, may himself provide meaningful consequences for the stutterer's behavior in the form of approval, disapproval, lack of understanding, or agreement.

The basic role of the clinician is to help modify the behavior (R) of the stutterer by arranging or providing consequences that immediately follow that behavior (all that is to the right of R in the diagram). The clinician has available to him those processes and events signified by Rf+, Rf−, Extinction, and Punishment. The effects of the various behaviors a clinician or his agent (parents, siblings, teachers) might emit as a consequence of the stutterer's behavior cannot be foretold, although we may make some educated guesses about the outcome. We can only determine the effects of our reactions during therapy by systematically and consistently engaging in a particular kind of behavior on a schedule, as a consequence of a predesignated behavior emitted by the stutterer.

The clinician may emit behaviors that convey support, approval, agreement, rejection and lack of acceptance, by smiling, saying "yes," "hm hm," scowling, or remaining silent. By tabulating what has happened to the behavior of the stutterer, we would then know more about the effects of our tactics.

Let us now take each of these consequent activities, define them, and see how they have been applied to the problem of stuttering.

Rf+ refers to a procedure known as *positive reinforcement*. If a response appears more frequently when followed by a particular event, the event that appears to increase the frequency of the response is called a positive reinforcer (provided that its removal reduces the frequency of the response.) An example might be the clinician doing something as simple as saying "good" or nodding and smiling in an approving manner immediately after the stutterer's report that he approached a feared talking situation, or after he deliberately modified some motor aspects of his stuttering.

The weakening or *extinction* of a response is brought about by removal of a reinforcer. For example, the therapist gives approval after each instance of stuttering in the early phases of therapy. By thus encouraging the stutterer to stutter freely, the therapist reinforces stuttering. Later in therapy, when he may want the stutterer to interrupt or modify his stuttering, the therapist withholds his approval. As a technique for weakening stuttering behavior, extinction may not be effective, because the response to be weakened (stuttering) must be under the control of the withheld reinforcer (approval). You cannot weaken through extinction what you do not control through reinforcement.

The introduction of some response-contingent events tends to interrupt or depress responses. This process is sometimes referred to as *punishment*. Punishment has probably been used in therapy more often than we like to think, and has been the subject of much research. Clinicians provide a ready model for the researcher to follow. When a clinician instructs a stutterer to reiterate a stuttered word, he may be asking the stutterer to punish himself by delaying his communicative message. Or when the clinician interrupts the stutterer who fails to do this, he himself may be punishing the stutterer. Disapproval can be communicated by facial expression, by head-shaking, by disagreeing, or merely by saying "no," or "you're wrong," or "I don't understand." Sometimes disapproval is communicated when the clinician is silent after the stutterer's behavior he thinks undesirable or that he wishes to weaken or suppress. These clinical behaviors can be thought to be aversive since a stutterer may increase in frequency those responses that tend to reduce or remove these events. The relation between responses and the consequences of terminating ongoing aversive events has been termed *negative reinforcement* (Rf—). Positive reinforcement (Rf+) and negative reinforcement (Rf—) imply a strengthening or an increased frequency of responses (R); while punishment and extinction imply a weakening or reduced frequency of responses. The effectiveness of these contingent consequent activities by the clinician can be determined by seeing whether the frequency of the responses they followed have systematically changed.

Table 2.1 suggests the form and content of some of those events that may come to control the stutterer's behavior during therapy. Some involve positive reinforcement and some involve negative reinforcement, while others illustrate mild punishment and extinction. Table 2.1 may be considered a skeleton outline of some of the things that clinicians do in therapy in order to manipulate the stutterer's problem.

TABLE 2.1. Possible Operant Paradigms That Characterize a Clinician's Manipulation of a Stutterer's Behavior During Therapy.

Occasion	Response	Consequence
Statement by therapist	*Response by stutterer*	*Response by clinician*
1. "Each time you stutter, say the word again." (instructional)	2. "O.K. I-I-I'll-I'll try."	3. "Fine, that's it." "You said the word 'I'll' again." (approval)
1. "Did you make the 5 telephone calls you said you would yesterday?" (question)	2. "No, I didn't have the time."	3. "Now just what does that mean, 'I didn't have the time.' " (disapproval)
1. "I think that today we ought to talk about some of the outside situations you are afraid to talk in." (orienting for content)	2. "Yes, sure, but first, did you happen to see that game on TV last night?"	3. Silence (extinction)

INFLUENCING
THE CLINICIAN'S BEHAVIOR

Just as the clinician may try to modify the stutterer's behavior during therapy in terms of certain contingent consequences, the clinician's behavior is also under some form of control. There are a number of variables that may operate to control the clinician's behavior during therapy. Many are elusive and difficult to analyze, such as our colleagues' opinions of our work, our previous training, our emotional needs at the moment, and perhaps, the behavior of the stutterer. We are going to focus only on the latter, with the recognition that these other factors are present and influence us.

Turning back to the diagram on page 23, we see that the same structure of events that operates in controlling the behavior of the stutterer operates in controlling the behavior of the clinician. This time, therefore, let the R in the center of the diagram stand for all the behaviors that clinicians have been observed to emit during therapy. These would include the various behaviors ascribed to clinicians earlier, such as asking questions, giving information, approving, disapproving. Just as there are occasions for the stutterer's behavior, there are also occasions that seem to evoke the clinician's behavior and consequent events that strengthen or weaken that behavior. Table 2.2 depicts some of these

TABLE 2.2. Possible Operant Paradigms That Characterize a Stutterer's Manipulation of Clinician's Responses During Therapy.

Occasion *Response by* *stutterer*	Response *Response by* *clinician*	Consequence *Response by* *stutterer*
1. An instant of stuttering	2. An instruction to the stutterer to modify his speech	3. Emission of appropriate modification (Rf+)
1. "I used to feel so helpless, but now I know I can control what I do." (self-description of a feeling)	2. "You mean that since you've been controlling your stuttering your feelings about yourself have changed." (interpretation correlating feeling and experience)	3. "No, that isn't what I meant exactly." (lack of acceptance of interpretation, punishment)
1. "What can I do— every time I start to talk on the phone, I freeze." (describing an event)	2. "What do you mean you freeze?" (asking for explanation)	3. "It's hard to explain —I press my lips together." (provides explanation) (Rf+)

events. Stuttering, for example, may be the occasion or the discriminative stimulus (S^D) for the clinician to instruct the stutterer in some form of modification of his speech response (R). The consequence the stutterer provided for the clinician's response could either strengthen or weaken the "instructing" behavior of the clinician. If the consequence is that the stutterer follows the clinician's instructions, "instruction responses" by the clinician would more than likely be strengthened, and become a common clinical behavior. But if the stutterer does not follow the instructions, we may see this type of response less frequently in therapy. Table 2.2 suggests how a clinician's behavior is also controlled through Rf+, Rf−, extinction, and punishment.

It should be apparent that the same event in therapy may have several functions, one or more functions for the stutterer, and other functions for the clinician. In general, almost all the events directly associated with the stutterer and the clinician are behavioral responses (R). Events like the air conditioner going on or the sunlight shining in the window are discounted. However, a verbal response may serve as a consequence for the response that preceded it and also as an evoking stimulus for the response that follows it, for both the stutterer and clinician. As an example, let us take a small sample dialogue from a clinical interview and speculate about the relationships which might be operating.

Response	*Functions*
1. Statement of clinician: "How was your speech at the meeting Friday night?"	S^D for stutterer's response 2
2. Statement by stutterer: "It was all right until they asked us to introduce ourselves. They were going in order and I was toward the end. As my turn approached I was getting tighter all the time."	Rf+ for clinician's response 1 S^D for clinician's response 3
3. Statement by clinician: "How did you say your name?"	Rf+ for stutterer's response 2 S^D for stutterer's response 4
4. Statement by stutterer: "I stuttered—I really messed up."	Rf+ for clinician's response 3 S^D for clinician's response 5
5. Statement by clinician: "How was your speech then the rest of the night?"	Rf+ for stutterer's response 4

As you can see, this is an ongoing dynamic process and not the S-R arrangement of discrete trials usually associated with conditioning. The verification of the functions listed in the right of the sample dialogue depends on systematic experimentations, wherein these events are systematically scheduled for occurrence during the interview, and their effects on the target responses are assessed. This then represents one of the most rigorous ways that the effectiveness of clinical behavior can be determined. Variations of this kind of analysis form the basis of the therapies described in this book.

THERAPY
AS OPERANT CONDITIONING:
A CONTROVERSY

There is a certain amount of controversy and debate surrounding the idea of therapy for stuttering being reduced to a process of conditioning. In this framework, we place the stutterer and the clinician in specific functional roles. One element of the controversy is the operant perception of the stutterer, whose various behaviors are our focus of attention. What he does and says becomes our target for manipulation and change. Another element is the role and function of the clinician, who provides antecedent events in the form of occasions for certain types of responses by the stutterer. The clinician also provides certain kinds of consequent events following the stutterer's behaviors, which he feels will bring about the desired therapeutic changes. Thus we have the events of therapy cast into the operant three-term paradigm of antecedent events → stutterer's responses → consequent events. This behavioral view of the processes of therapy has very vocal and tenacious proponents and opponents.

Very likely, the most serious and profound opposition to an operant approach to stuttering therapy is that it deals solely with observable behavior. This focus on observable behavior probably, in part, reflects the experimental, laboratory heritage of scientific rigor and operational descriptiveness from which operant conditioning techniques derive. Operant conditioning has an ancestry of controlled animal research in the laboratory. It is only recently that clinicians have begun to explore the possibilities of selectively applying operant techniques to therapy.

In the laboratory, the responses to be manipulated must be designated and defined in advance, and the things that the experimenter does must be precisely described and scheduled for occurrence. Focus is on the observable events associated with the behavior of the stutterer as well as the behavior of the clinician. The precise quantification of these activities rather than the reporting of casual impressions is necessary. Such quantitative behavioral description should enable a consistent replication of an experimental arrangement so that we may ultimately draw some decisive conclusions about our ability to experimentally modify behavior under controlled conditions.

The practice of designating in advance relevant responses by the stutterer and the clinician, of categorizing and tabulating different types of responses, and restricting ourselves to only certain types of reactions may be suspect in the clinical situation. From the standpoint of therapy, these activities can be perceived as closing the door on a number of clinical styles and on a number of theoretical conceptual models of stuttering. For example, clinicians like to think that they are dealing with the whole person, rather than some fragment of behavior. Also, they like to feel that they are free to deal with anything they deem important, as it arises, rather than only with what has been designated as a target response. Clinicians also strive to retain their freedom to respond in a number of ways to the behaviors of a stutterer rather than in a limited fashion which has been spelled out by some previously designated contingency arrangement. From the conditioning point of view, these kinds of freedoms constitute inconsistency. Not consistently adhering to a schedule of contingencies usually leads to unsuccessful conditioning, and at best, difficulties in documenting successful or unsuccessful outcomes. If there were only one item of information for the clinician to glean from the operant laboratories, it would deal with the effects of certain schedules of contingent events and the need for their consistent application. Of course, for the clinician, being programmed to a schedule of activity minimizes human judgment. Judgment is a valuable possession of the clinician even though it may be fraught with errors and inconsistencies. Perhaps some compromise is possible between clinical judgment on the one hand and programmed consistency on the other. It is the age-old problem of relevance versus reliability. The wise clinician knows when it is time to shift gears from a consistent but less relevant activity, to one that may intuitively seem valid and important during a clinical interview. But this same wise clinician should exercise these judgments carefully. Such shifts in emphasis of content, or changes in his behavior mean he is temporarily (or permanently) terminating a particular line of thought or conditioning arrangement in which he and the stutterer may have invested considerable time and thought.

Another legitimate question raised by clinicians has to do with the conditioner's preoccupation with frequency counts of behavior as the most significant kind of information to be dealt with. Clinicians know that often the single, initial, or infrequent occurrence of a particular behavior may be more significant clinically than reoccurrences of the same behavior, or than hundreds of occurrences of another type of behavior. They may well ask how this kind of single, initial, or infrequent event can be accounted for. For example, is the first statement by a stutterer that reflects insight or describes a correlate to his stuttering equivalent to fifty similar statements later? Of course, appropriately designed research that systematically relates these kinds of single, initial, or infrequent events to changes in overt stuttering could provide the answers. These questions raised by clinicians should not be ruled out or dismissed as nonresearchable clinical events or as unreasonable questions.

Clinicians also justifiably question the social carryover of what looks like a gadget-oriented laboratory demonstration. How much of the change in stuttering that is observed in the controlled operant laboratory is meaningful outside the laboratory? It appears that the clinician and the researcher should separate laboratory demonstration experiments with their focus and goals from operant-based therapy and its focus and goals. It should be noted that the experimentalist is not necessarily interested in demonstrating long-term effects of his experimental manipulation of stuttering. His primary interest may have been in discovering contingencies for manipulating the frequency of stuttering under highly controlled conditions. Thus, it is not reasonable to expect information about carryover from such research. At the same time, however, the clinician should be alert to the possible application to therapy of the experimentalist's tactics as well as to the limitations. In other words, reducing stuttering frequency in a laboratory is not the same as treating an individual who stutters.

What of the private side of stuttering, which most of us agree is also a part of the problem? It appears that for operantly oriented people, stuttering is merely the frequency of its overt occurrence and nothing more. The concepts of operant behavior do not deal, to the clinician's satisfaction, with such things as the stutterer's attitudes, feelings, and emotions. The emotional forces that operate in all of us (stutterers as well), and that may be significant factors in the origins and directions of our behavior, have only been minimally dealt with in the operant framework. Most of the time, emotions are viewed as processes that interefere with operant behavior and are of a different general nature. However, emotions may also be instrumentally controlled and serve as a positive directing force in therapy as well as in many of our other interpersonal experiences. Most of us have seen a stutterer who at the outset of a therapy session appeared depressed and predicted that "today will be a bad day." We may also have seen some stutterers who stutter more when happy and excited, or who stutter more frequently when angry or depressed. The relation between a particular emotional state or mood and the occurrence of stuttering is poorly understood.

There have been some attempts to control emotional states. For example, certain indices of emotion (heart rate, blood pressure, pulse, and GSR) have been brought under operant control. In addition, the efficacy of using drugs for controlling moods and feelings is now being investigated. At this time, however, neither the operant control of emotions nor the administration of drugs has become a technique for helping the stutterer.

Finally, in a more personal vein, many clinicians do not like to think of themselves as manipulators of someone else's behavior; they prefer to believe that the person is helping himself, directing himself, and self-actualizing his potential.

These are all serious comments of importance to the operant point of view. Although many are critical issues and require examination, mere recitation by clinicians does not relieve these clinicians of the responsibility for asking the same questions about their own current activities. The same tests of effectiveness and description of procedures called for in the operant framework can be applied as validly to current clinical procedures with stutterers.

The operantly oriented workers, clinicians, and researchers alike recognize that the work on this subject must be viewed, for the most part, as research, and not as tried-and-true therapy procedures. This recognition is not a response to the critical comments that have been leveled at them, but rather it characterizes their view of their basic mission—to develop valid and effective therapy procedures based on logical principles of behavior modification, supported by reliable and valid research data.

This research has resulted in a number of suggestions and speculations about the prevention of stuttering and therapy for stuttering. However, there has been very little published information about clinical application. The little published information about operantly based therapy has contained only fragmentary data about social carryover (either short- or long-term) of the behavioral changes noted in the "experimental therapy" session. However, we should point out that the lack of information on this subject is no worse a state of affairs than the situation surrounding more traditional therapies for stuttering, where this information is also lacking. We should all seek to clean our own glass houses in this regard. For the most part, the researchers have left the clinical application of their research to the artistry of the clinician. It is no longer a question of whether the clinician is a manipulator of behavior. We are definitely involved in trying to change or help the stutterer to change the way he talks. It is now a question of how good a manipulator we clinicians can become. Unless stuttering is reduced or eliminated from the speaker's way of behaving, everything else that may happen to a stutterer is of questionable validity and of questionable value, insofar as therapy for stuttering is concerned. Therapy for stuttering means just that—therapy for stuttering. Unless we restrict ourselves to dealing with observable behaviors, we may find ourselves manipulating only our own theories about stuttering with little reference but much inference about the stutterer's stuttering behavior.

Operant applications to stuttering do not have to be limited to electromechanical laboratory demonstrations. The problems of therapy require that this work should be extended to the field and social milieu of the stutterer, and that the real-life encounters of the stutterer should be brought into this framework in a systematic way. To encourage this attitude further, we underscore the fact that there really is no operant conditioning theory of stuttering, rather that operant conditioning suggests a way of relating a series of events to one another (i.e., antecedent event → stuttering response → consequent event) that may be productive in affecting the development, maintenance, and therapeutic reduction of stuttering.

It is also apparent that, insofar as therapy is concerned, operant conditioning provides some strategies for behavior modification and nothing more. These strategies need to be filled in with some content. It should be clear that a strategy of manipulation does not tell us what is to be manipulated. The specific forms of the events to be manipulated in an operant framework derive from the bona fide content theories of stuttering (i.e., forms of dysfluency, thematic content of language, self-perceptions, anticipation behavior, avoidance behavior, conflict behavior), as long as these concepts can be placed in relation to one another as observable events.

One of the most serious indictments proffered by the advocates of operant conditioning and behavior modification concerns the final goals of therapy. Unlike others, we feel that stutterers should not be asked to accept their stuttering, to learn to live with their stuttering, and to modify it into more socially acceptable forms. The goal for many of the operant and behavior modification oriented workers is speech that is free from stuttering. This goal may or may not be realistic—only research and clinical application will provide an answer—but this difference in goals is basic regarding behavior in general, stuttering dynamics in particular, and the nature of therapy.

SUMMARY

The principles and concepts of operant conditioning emerged from behavioral studies of animals in the laboratory. So successful were these laboratory activities in terms of training, teaching, and controlling the behavior of animals that potential applications to human behavior could not be ignored. Such applications raise many issues. Most prominent are the equating of man with the laboratory animal and the control of a person without his being aware of that control. Talking chimpanzees notwithstanding, we believe that man's linguistic capacity invalidates any claim that the laboratory animal is his equal. In addition, we abhor any invidious forms of behavioral control. We are, however, interested in exploring the efficacy of operant principles applied to the management of stuttering. In this chapter we began that exploration. We suggested the manner in which the behaviors exhibited by stutterers and clinicians could be defined in operant terminology and assigned to the respective components of the operant model. In subsequent chapters we expand upon this application and exploration.

3

....

The Evaluation
of Stuttering

SOME ASSUMPTIONS
AND GENERAL PRINCIPLES
OF EVALUATION

Most of us would agree that there are several goals to be achieved in an evaluation of stuttering. One goal is to describe the problem in terms of the stutterer and the various ways that he may express or manifest his problem. This description of the problem should include the circumstances and contexts of its expression, such as the people, situations, and various other occasions and consequences for the stutterer's behavior. It should include the actions and events that appear to maintain stuttering as well as those associated with being relatively fluent. Second, an evaluation should provide a prognosis for therapy. We should be able to make an educated prediction whether or not a stutterer will benefit from our therapy. Third, an evaluation should provide information for developing therapy strategies. These goals are assumed to underlie all evaluations, whether for stuttering or for any type of behavioral problem.

What clinicians might not agree on are some additional goals, such as the importance of determining etiology, the scope and nature of the behavior to be described, and the frame of reference or dimensions that are employed in describing the problem. It is also almost certain that we will disagree on how we should go about conducting an evaluation.

Given these assumptions of our common goals, it follows that there should be a clear functional relation among: (1) our theory of relevant and related events in the problem of stuttering; (2) our evaluative transactions and focus (those things that are evaluated) ; and (3) our clinical management and therapy (those things that are going to be attended to in therapy) . In others words, the way we view the problem dictates what we evaluate. And in turn, what we evaluate should reflect the issues we plan to deal with in therapy.

Therefore, if our view of the stuttering problem involves the importance of interpersonal relations between the young child and his parents, and as a result, if our therapy is programmed to deal with such complicated issues, then the evaluative focus should include considerable attention to such interpersonal relationships. On the other hand, if our view of the stuttering problem involves the stutterer's self-image and perceptions of himself, and our therapy therefore is designed to deal with those issues, then as a result, our evaluative transactions should focus on the stutterer's self-image.

It is not our purpose to compare, contrast, and illustrate similarities and differences between traditional clinical procedures and procedures associated with an operant point of view. But it is essential to point out many of the historical derivations and departures of operant tactics. In many instances the history of traditional theory, the methods of observation, tactics for gathering information, and inferences and interpretations breathe life and form into the applications of descriptive behaviorism to stuttering.

A traditional evaluation of a stuttering problem, with its goals of describing an individual's speech, social, and emotional behavior, of correlating the speaker with his environment, of prognosis, and of planning therapy, has employed such tactics as:

1. Observing the stutterer and his family.
2. Developing a social and developmental case history by interviewing the stutterer and various members of his family.
3. Administering tests.

From these clinical tactics of testing, interviewing, observing, and history-taking, the clinician tries to put together the stutterer's story. The chronicle of his life's historical events, when combined with his current life system and test data, enables the clinician to draw inferences and conclusions relevant to the goals of the evaluation (description, prognosis, planning) and their relation to therapy. Each tactic and evaluative activity and each evaluative goal should be related to the goals and processes of therapy.

There are a number of variations of this basic evaluation model that depend on emphasis, but for the most part the goals are similar. For example, in the usual psychiatric setting, a social worker may obtain a social case history, a psychologist may administer and interpret psychological tests, and, together with a psychiatrist, a decision is made about the appropriateness of psychotherapy. The medical model of cause and effect in which stuttering is viewed as a symptom of some underlying emotional problem is applied.

In the context of client-centered counseling, there is a departure from some of these procedures. Case histories are not taken and tests are not administered. The vehicle for deciding on the appropriateness of this type of therapy is the clinical interview. If therapy is initiated, the counselor is not influenced by any preconceived or stereotyped categories of psychological information, and can respond to the current material that is important at the moment the stutterer presents it to the counselor. However, it should be pointed out that these counselors are programmed to respond one way to emotional material and emotional expressions during an interview, and in another way to intellectual material and expressions. In effect, the stutterer is directed to talk more about some things and less about others, through the timely and strategic reflections of the counselor (Rogers, 1942). The focus is less on any one presenting symptom and more on basic emotional (or cognitive) processes that interfere with the stutterer's realization of his full human potential. Here, too, stuttering is viewed as a symptom of a more basic problem.

More recently, reciprocal inhibition and desensitization therapy have been applied to the stuttering problem (Wolpe, 1958; Lanyon, 1969; Damste, 1970). Although this may involve the usual history-taking and testing procedures, the crucial aspect of evaluation here involves the reporting of anxiety hierarchies. The stutterer is asked to describe various situations that elicit anxiety, and to rate each situation in terms of anxiety level. These hierarchies become the nucleus around which therapy is organized, and the stutterer's anxiety is systematically manipulated in an attempt to reduce stuttering. Again, stuttering is viewed as a symptom of something else, in this case, anxiety about talking.

These examples of approaches to evaluation differ from one another and resemble one another. Each uses interviewing as a vehicle for sampling behavior. Each assumes that stuttering is a symptom of something more basic to the individual and that this something else is the thing to be evaluated and dealt with in therapy. Each seems to relate theory, evaluation, and management in a direct way. However, each approach does not involve the administration of formal psychological tests, nor does each involve the accumulation of a client's life history.

The illustration of the variations in evaluation tactics may put into perspective the evaluative tactics associated with an operant-based approach. At best, all evaluative procedures can be viewed as tactics that attempt to obtain representative samples of the stutterer's problems, based on small sampling techniques. The tests, the direct observations, the clinical interviews and case histories, are sampling devices that can provide the information necessary for describing, prognosticating, and planning about the stuttering problem.

Since the behavioristic view of stuttering explicitly states that stuttering is not a symptom, but is separately manipulable behavior, the focus during evaluation is on those factors that enter into its manipulation—namely, the observable speech responses themselves (fluent and stuttered) of the stutterer, and the antecedent and consequent events that control their occurrence. It should be recognized, however, that the speech responses of the stutterer may not be the only behaviors that are significant to the problem of stuttering. Homme (1965) has coined the term "coverants" for covert behaviors that can also be made public and observable. Through introspective reporting by the stutterer these typically private behaviors can be made available as legitimate target responses that can be viewed within the antecedent-consequent paradigms of operant conditioning. This expanded view of the problem as more than merely the overt frequency of certain types of speech responses broadens the horizons of operant therapy considerably. With coverants in mind, the problem can also include feeling states, self-images, emotional excitement, attitudes, as long as representations of such phenomena are made observable and the circumstances for their emission can be analyzed and verified.

The thrust of such operant-based evaluations is to generate *base rates* of target behaviors. Base rates are the frequency of a pertinent behavior over a given amount of time, or over a given number of responses, i.e., the number of words stuttered for every 100 words uttered, or the number of words stuttered per minute. Base rates like tests and case history taking involve obtaining representative samples of behavior that are significant to the problem. In order to maximize their representativeness, these base rates ideally should be obtained under circumstances that begin to resemble those situations that an individual stutterer encounters in his everyday life. Usually, base rates are obtained in limited stimulus circumstances, and like other sampling devices and test interpretations, a small sample of the total is assumed to be representative and therefore predictive of the stutterer's behaviors in those circumstances that were not sampled. The goal is to develop a behavioral profile of the stutterer before therapy. The profile should describe the problem behaviorally (operant and coverant), tell us what behaviors need attention during therapy, and give us a base against which the effects of therapy can be measured.

Here again is an example of evaluation tactics that do not involve obtaining a case history or administering tests, but instead involve arranging for direct observation of current behavior. The tactics may or may not involve interviewing as a vehicle for making such observations. They could range from asking a stutterer to tell stories about pictures he is looking at to observing an actual social interaction between the stutterer and his parents. Specific evaluation tactics will be described in a later section of this chapter. However, in relation to the other models of evaluation already described, the operant-based model represents another variation involving a functional relation among the view of the problem, the evaluation procedures, and later therapeutic transactions. Its goals also are a description of the problem, discovering current maintaining factors, and planning therapy. These general principles of evaluation underlie the various specific evaluation transactions to be described, and are at the core of the many different ways evaluations may be carried out.

SPECIFIC EVALUATION PROCEDURES

The operant paradigm for analyzing behavior contains three elements, namely (1) the specific behaviors under consideration (speech, social, emotional, etc.) ; (2) the occasions for their emission; and (3) the consequent events affecting their frequency of occurrence. It therefore follows that our system for evaluating the problem will focus on verifying a series of hypothesized relationships among (1) the stutterer's (or nonstutterer's, in the case of normal dysfluency) speech responses, both fluent and dysfluent; (2) the events that immediately precede these speech responses; and (3) the events that immediately follow these speech responses. In addition to speech responses, our theoretical point of view about the nature of the stuttering problem may require us to observe in a similar fashion other target behaviors, such as the content of the stutterer's remarks about himself (i.e., his helplessness, his victimization), anticipatory behavior, eye contact, or vacillating conflict behavior. The original hypotheses about these relations among antecedent events, target responses, and consequent events derive from observation of the person's behaviors under a number of different circumstances. Therefore, the first step in developing the evaluation and in making judgments about a person's speech is to arrange for a series of observations of his behaviors; and from these observations to fill in the three elements of the operant paradigm, namely, the occasions for target responses, the responses themselves, and the consequent events that follow them. Such observations of the total episode will provide us with the behavioral profiles that will help us to make judgments about the appropriateness of professional intervention, and the nature of that intervention, if it is dictated.

In the typical clinical situation, our first contact with a stutterer (child or adult) is in a quasi-interview, conversational setting during which we have an opportunity to observe the form, frequency, and duration of instances of dysfluency. We can also observe associated behaviors and mannerisms that may be related to talking, such as eye blinking, head shaking, tongue protruding, and so on. This is usually a casual situation during which the focus is on obtaining a sample of the speaker's behavior, with little or no attention to antecedent and consequent events. An analysis of the total behavioral paradigm is not quite so casual an undertaking. First, of course, we have to decide in advance what antecedent and consequent events we wish to observe as they may function in determining the emission of fluent and dysfluent speech. This decision more than likely is based on our past experiences with children and adults who are stutterers; our knowledge of the factors that affect the occurrence of dysfluency; our familiarity with the research literature; and the information provided us by the subject speaker and members of his family who have had opportunities to observe his speaking behavior. Our task then is to observe the frequency of pertinent target behaviors during a number of occasions that resemble the speaker's real life encounters. These occasions may vary in importance or significance from stutterer to stutterer. Our past experience tells us that stuttering may vary with the people being spoken to, with the speaking situation, with the size of the audience, with the topic of conversation, with the speaker's excitement, with the nature of the social interaction, with the function and form of the speaker's linguistic output, with the length of utterance, and with the significance of the speaking situation to the speaker's life system. These all constitute occasions for speaking, either fluently or dysfluently. The clinician's task is to arrange to sample the speaker's behavior in a systematic way during these occasions to determine if in fact the speaker's dysfluency does vary with variations of the properties of these occasions. Some of these occasions may be relatively simple to arrange while others could become quite complicated and involve special equipment. Table 3.1 lists each of these occasions and suggests ways for sampling the speaker's behavior.

The occasions and sampling tactics that appear in Table 3.1 are only guidelines and suggestions for events that may be significant to an individual stutterer's problem. The techniques for determining whether

TABLE 3.1. Suggested Occasions and Tactics for Evaluating Stuttering.

Occasion Variable	Sampling Tactic
Audience size	Have the speaker talk first to one person, then to two, and increase the size of the audience up to seven people, adding one person each time. There is no fixed amount of time for each condition, but probably a minimum of five minutes each would be appropriate. To determine the reliability of such information, the entire procedure should be replicated.
Specific people	Ask the stutterer (or members of his family if it is a child) to tell you the names of three people he stutters the most with and three people with whom he is consistently fluent. With portable recording equipment, arrange to obtain the cooperation of these six people to obtain a short sample of the stutterer's speech during conversation with them.
Different talking situations	Ask the stutterer or members of his family to indicate those situations that he stutters the most in and those that he is usually most fluent in (three of each type) and arrange to tape record the speaker talking in those situations. We are referring to such situations as talking on the telephone, asking directions, giving information (the situations listed in the Trotter-Bergman Level of Situational Difficulty Scale, 1957).
	Of particular importance may be the stutterer's home environment situation and/or school situation. These two situations should be sampled in addition to the other situations indicated.
Competition for talking time (interruption)	During an interview or play situation with a child (in a conversational setting) systematically schedule a series of interruptions of the speaker's verbal responses.
Length of utterance	In an interview situation ask the stutterer questions that require verbal responses of increasing length in a progression from short to long, i.e.,
	Five questions requiring a "yes" or "no" answer.
	Five questions requiring a two-word response, as in naming objects in a picture.
	A sentence completion task requiring a progression of longer responses (one word to completion, then two words to completion, then three words to completion, etc.).
	A standardized interview of a question-and-answer type that systematically includes responses of varying lengths, i.e.,
	Your name address age birth date
	Analyze length of utterances in free conversation relative to dysfluency, without necessarily structuring in any systematic way the length of the stutterer's response, with the assumption that various lengths will occur in a free conversational situation (unless the stutterer has learned to avoid emitting those utterance lengths associated with stuttering).

TABLE 3.1. (Continued)

Occasion Variable	Sampling Tactic
Topic of conversation	In an interview situation direct the conversation for certain amounts of time to various topics such as home life, occupation, goals and aspirations, speaking, social activities.
Emotional excitement	Ask the stutterer to describe in detail and to re-create as accurately as possible instances when he was happy, angry, afraid, depressed, hostile, relaxed.
	Related to the above, if the equipment is available, obtain physiological data such as heart rate, GSR, EMG, EKG, as correlates to the verbal material associated with various moods.
Social and verbal interactions	Arrange to observe (in the clinic or home) an actual short interaction between the speaker and members of his family (mother, father, wife, children, siblings). Tape record (video and/or audio) for later analysis of global nature of the interaction as well as specific events that precede and follow dysfluencies. Categories of verbal interaction have been developed in previous research by Egolf et al. (1972) and Kasprisin-Burrelli et al. (1972) and are available for use.
Linguistic units and functions	During an interview, systematically have the stutterer answer questions, give directions, explain a concept, justify an opinion, correct a comment by the clinician, confirm, negate, ask a question, give a command, describe a state of affairs, respond to rejection and hostility.
Time pressure	During an interview systematically vary the amount of time provided for a verbal response by the speaker. This can be done more systematically by using a tachistoscope for presenting a stimulus for varying amounts of time and providing a payoff for responses within certain time limits provided, or more simply with a time signal (noise, bell, light, hand signal, etc.).

these occasions are important are also only suggestions. It is clear that clinicians can approach these tasks in a number of ways. However, the purpose is to arrange as much as possible for direct observation rather than to depend solely on verbal reports and memory, or on tests that may be quite remote from the behavior under consideration.

When we have made systematic observations and noted the frequencies of target responses, we can then start making some judgments about the speech of the speaker.

A major issue in the evaluation of speech fluency is deciding whether, in fact, we are faced with stuttering. We usually encounter the problem of differentiating stuttering from other types of dysfluency in the preschool age child, although there are occasions when we encounter this problem in adults.

There are three types of dysfluency that should be distinguished from one another in the young child. One of these has come to be known as normal developmental dysfluency. A second is dysfluency that is a response to unusual environmental stress, while the third is dysfluency that is associated with the problem of stuttering. The differentiation among these three types of dysfluency is extremely important, because each type has separate implications for therapeutic intervention (Shames, 1968).

When we use the term "type of dysfluency," we are not referring to differences in the forms of dysfluency, such as whole word repetition versus part word repetition versus interjections and pauses. Classifying a child's speech as normally dysfluent, as dysfluent in response to environmental stress, or as stuttering is extremely difficult if the classification is based solely on the form of the dysfluent speech because there is so much similarity and overlap among these three classifications. Both stutterers and nonstutterers are dysfluent and fluent, and very often in highly similar ways. Therefore, the process of differentiation must include an analysis of additional factors. These additional factors include the following:

1. A descriptive history of how the speech dysfluencies have changed in form, frequency, and circumstances.
2. Observations of the consistency of the dysfluencies.
3. The occasions for the emission of dysfluency.
4. The current form and frequency.
5. The reactions of listeners, including the alleged dysfluent speaker himself.

Ideally, information about these factors should be based on the direct observations of the evaluator. However, certain of these items (such as item 1, the history of change) can only be evaluated through the observations and memories of people who have been a part of that history, usually parents, relatives, and the speaker. It would appear, therefore, that certain types of information are appropriately learned from historical interviews while other types of information ought to be based on direct observation.

NORMAL DYSFLUENCY*

When parents decide whether a child's dysfluency is normal or not, they have an idea of the way most children talk. Obviously, this idea

---

* Much of the material in this section appeared in Shames (1968). Used by permission of the publishers, W. B. Saunders.

varies greatly, depending on the adult's experience, so that different listeners evaluate the speech behavior of a child differently. A child one listener considers abnormally dysfluent may be considered normally dysfluent by another.

Davis (1939, 1940) and Winitz (1961) have suggested that speech dysfluencies like repetitions, prolongations, interjections, and pauses occur relatively often in young children. Repetitions have been the most frequently observed form, as the repetition of codified speech is a part of the child's repertoire by the age of two years. These repetitions may be of whole words, parts of words, or several words or phrases. It is of interest that the repetitions of whole words and of several words or a phrase are more often thought characteristic of the normal developmental process, while syllable repetition or part word repetition more often results in a diagnosis of stuttering.

It seems that the breaking up of the rhythm of the utterance of a single word constitutes a greater departure from the basic rhythm of language than the rhythm breaks associated with whole word and phrase repetitions. The symbolic meaning of an utterance and its intelligibility may be only minimally distorted in whole word and phrase repetition, while these qualities are seriously impaired in syllable repetition. These factors may be potent in deciding that syllable repetition constitutes a dysfluency problem, while whole word and phrase repetition are considered normal dysfluencies. As a result, speech clinicians have become alerted to watching for the occurrence of part word repetition as a danger signal, while whole word and phrase repetitions may often be evaluated as normal in the absence of unusual environmental circumstances.

The conditions associated with the original emission and early development of nonfluencies in the speech of infants are still obscure and in need of detailed observation. It is possible that the repetitions observed in what is called dysfluency in later life may be related to the vocal behavior of infants during their early speech development, such as babbling and syllable chaining. Winitz's observations of repetitions in the vocal behavior of infants offer data to support such a hypothesis.

It is also possible that the physiologic characteristics of the human organism are such that speech dysfluencies are a "wired-in" characteristic. Structured speech, after all, is an adjunctive function of organs having other basic biologic functions, and as such, speech appears within the limitations imposed by these other functions. We must pause and hesitate, if only to inhale. Thinking of speech dysfluency as a function of a physiologic predisposition of humans may suggest that dysfluency should be expected to occur and, therefore, that it has a general aura of normality about it. However, this is not a necessary or requisite conclusion. Although the physiologic restrictions imposed may in fact result in the fundamental rhythms and rates of speech that are a part of language, logically these physiologic constraints would appear in the forms of normal pauses and hesitations in speech. It is difficult to connect them with any of the various forms of speech repetitions. These repetitions, on the contrary, appear to be acquired or learned responses, some of which may constitute problems and some of which may not.

Let us now look at a few illustrations of what may be considered normal dysfluency. It has been observed that the speaker's verbal behavior varies in response to such listener actions as looking, nodding, smiling, speaking, or doing something for the speaker. We infer that these consequent activities reinforce the speaker, because we observe that the speaker continues to speak as long as these activities continue. We also observe that the speaker's behavior diminishes in strength when these activities are no longer forthcoming.

It is possible to view the repetition response as a special class of verbal response, whose initial appearance may have a basis foreign to its development as dysfluency (Shames and Sherrick, 1963). For example, a speaker may repeat a statement in order to make sure that it has been heard correctly. After several occasions of such repetition, the speaker is "reinforced for repetitions," and on future occasions the repetitions may increase in number.

Speakers often compose, edit, and prompt themselves while speaking. Staccato speech units of varying sizes and dimensions are punctuated by pauses, during which it is thought that the processes of composition and editing go on. The emission of speech and its composition and editing appear to be almost simultaneous activities. As a speaker hears and feels himself speak, he monitors what he hears and feels. Sometimes he changes and corrects certain aspects of his utterances, such as his articulation, his pitch, his rhythm, or his combination of phonemes. These changes and corrections are often heard as short repetitions of sounds or syllables or words. It is felt that these composing and editing processes are primarily a result of the continuous feedback and monitoring of speech behavior. These processes may be among the prime factors in the dysfluencies of young children, who are still linguistically immature and actively involved in developing language skills.

Related to the processes of editing and composing is yet another possible function of speech dysfluencies. This is the function of obtaining and holding the attention of a listener. The composing process may also be partly under the control of the attending listener. As long as "attending" continues, composition and speech emission continue. When attending is withdrawn, speech and presumably composition diminish. It is possible that the repetition response may serve to hold the attention of the listener during composition. Therefore, while a child is composing, he may emit repetitions to fill the silence produced by pauses for composition, and to prevent the listener from interpreting those pauses as cues for speaking. Such repeated interjections as "uh," "ah," and "um um" are frequently encountered in the speech of adults as well as children. In fact, often when such repetitions to fill pauses during composition are not emitted by speakers, such pauses can be mistakenly identified as signals to the listener that the speaker has terminated that particular utterance. If the listener then chooses to speak, he may be embarrassed to find himself in the role of an interrupter.

From this discussion and the illustrative processes suggested as being involved in normal dysfluency, several concluding hypotheses are offered:

1. Pauses in speech appear to be events toward which the human being is physiologically predisposed. Such pauses are often thought of as speech dysfluencies but they are more likely to function as accommodations to the basic rhythms and limitations of our physiological systems.
2. One general class of speech dysfluency behavior, speech repetitions (sound, syllable, word, and phrase), appears to be learned.
3. As learned behavior, normal speech repetitions are not randomly emitted, but are controlled in an orderly system through various environmental circumstances.
4. Some of the circumstances, processes, and functions suggested as being involved in normal dysfluency are:
   a. obtaining a listener's attention;
   b. composing and editing speech and language responses;
   c. filling silences created by pauses to prevent the listener from speaking.
5. Normal dysfluency does not require professional intervention.

DYSFLUENCY ASSOCIATED
WITH ENVIRONMENTAL PRESSURE

A decision about the normality of dysfluency involves the judgment that professional intervention is necessary to modify the speech behavior of the child. This judgment is based in part on the attitudes of the child's listeners and in part on the speech emitted by the child. However, such a decision for the professional also involves an evaluation of the environmental factors that may influence the child's speech. The abnormality is not viewed with reference only to the speech behavior of the child, but, as importantly, with reference to the child's environment. The abnormality may be in the events going on around the child, to which the child may be reacting normally. In this sense the child's dysfluency may be considered a normal reaction to an abnormal environment. Professional intervention to modify the child's speech under these circumstances is not necessarily directed toward the child, but rather toward modifying the factors in his environment that influence his emission of speech dysfluencies. Like normal dysfluency, dysfluency that is related to environmental pressure also appears to be primarily learned, orderly, and under the control of variables that can be specified in the environment.

The research by Davis (1939, 1940), which suggested that certain forms of dysfluency were normal and to be expected, contained some additional and important information about the circumstances for the emission of dysfluencies. Davis observed that repetitions, which were the commonest form of dysfluency, seemed to be related to getting attention, directing someone else's activities, trying to gain an object, coercion, seeking status, giving and seeking information, criticizing, seeking a privilege, or trying to obtain social acceptance. It is interesting to note that nearly all of these occasions involve a type of verbal behavior expressed in the interrogative or imperative moods. Skinner (1957) suggests that this type of verbal behavior is controlled by a listener's consequent reactions to such utterances on the occasions of specific states of deprivation for the child, or on the occasions of aversive stimulation (stimulus situations that appear to make the child uncomfortable or that the child avoids, withdraws from, tries to terminate, or dislikes).

Typically, the listener does something for the speaker or gives something to the speaker. The listener's behavior can increase the likelihood of a particular form of verbal behavior by the speaker on future occasions of similar aversive stimulation or deprivation. An example is the young child who falls and is hurt or becomes frightened. He shouts "Mommy, Mommy, I'm hurt, I'm hurt, up, up!" The child's mother comes and lifts him and soothes him. The child has indicated to his mother the behavior that will "reinforce" his utterance. In the future, if the child wants his mother to lift him up he may emit the same form of verbal behavior. Davis's observations suggest that a relation between repetition responses and occasions of aversive stimulation or states of deprivation should be studied.

Clinically, one must judge whether a particular state of deprivation or aversive situation resulting in speech dysfluency should be reduced or modified, or whether such a situation is a part of everyday living. If it is the latter, then some speech clinicians directly involve the child in desensitization activities (Van Riper, 1954; Egland, 1954; Van Riper, 1973) which gradually make him more tolerant of these pressures. This is done by experimentally withdrawing or reducing pressures and gradually reintroducing them without precipitating speech dysfluency. Eventually this new tolerance for pressure is systematically generalized to the child's environment at home and to the pressures he encounters in everyday life. This, of course, is a situation in which the speech dysfluency of the child is a function of his intolerance for pressure rather than of an abnormal, highly pressured environment.

There may, however, be times when, even under normal environmental circumstances, a decision is made to reduce normal pressures temporarily, to the point where they are nonfunctional. In such instances, few if any demands are made upon the child as a temporary measure, during a particularly critical stage of speech dysfluency. Such clinical strategies are often difficult to implement in the complex system of a family or social community. They also have to be closely monitored and gradually terminated. It should be recognized that such strategies, if not employed properly, run the risk of begetting a spoiled child who develops unrealistic views and maladaptive behavior relative to his role in society and the demands and constraints he should expect from society.

It should also be pointed out that the demanding behavior of a child on the occasion of physical or social deprivation or aversive stimulation is usually strengthened in a somewhat haphazard, variable manner by parents. Often the demands of a child are satisfied at the convenience of the adult. Such a variable pattern of reinforcement may accomplish two things. One of these is to establish the child's behavior so strongly that it may be resistant to extinction. Data from experimental behavior laboratories suggest that such is the case for variable interval schedules of reinforcement. Second, this pattern of reinforcement may result in sustaining the social deprivation operating for the child at a consistently high level, thereby increasing the probability of a particular response that has reduced a deprivation in the past. These factors can become active variables in speech dysfluency if speech repetitions become connected with the variable reinforcement of these demands. It appears possible that if these connections occur frequently, the speech repetitions will appear in greater strength, since they are being reinforced on the same schedule as the child's verbal behavior of demanding, commanding, and asking questions. An example might be the parent who delays responding to a child's first utterance because of the inconvenience of doing so. The child may then repeat the utterance several times, until the repetition becomes undesirable to the parent. The parent finally comes to the child's rescue and does whatever he has demanded, perhaps unaware that he is not only doing something for his child but is also teaching him to repeat.

If we extend this example to consider some future behavior of the parent, we may eventually see some etiological relations among (1) the inconvenience of responding to his child's demands; (2) a connection between the child's speech repetition and this inconvenience, resulting in the repetitions becoming an aversive event for the parent; (3) the reinforcement of speech repetitions along with the reinforcement of the demanding behavior of the child, as the parent attempts to terminate this aversive "nagging" behavior of the child; and (4) the later punishment of the child's aversive speech repetitions, because they may occur not only when the child is making demands on his parents, but at any time. These relations are often seen in the development of stuttering.

Another function of the speech repetition may be found in relation to aversive stimuli. A child may show avoidance of certain unpleasant conditions by his verbal behavior. The speech repetition response may be used to postpone or avoid aversive painful conditions known to be associated with a forthcoming portion of the verbal response. For example, if aversive consequences follow a lie or the admission of responsibility for a socially unacceptable act, the child may be observed trying to postpone or avoid that crucial aversive part of his utterance by repeating an interjection or repeating a word or a phrase before such a response.

A final illustration of a commonly encountered environmental pressure associated with dysfluency, which is usually amenable to professional intervention, is the problem of competition for talking time in the home. Children typically seem to learn quite early that two people in conversation do not talk at exactly the same time. The silence of the conversational partner serves as the occasion for one's own speech, while the sound of the partner's voice calls for one to be silent and listen. However, sometimes the conversational partner's silence is only a short pause while he is composing his response and is not meant to be a cue for the child to speak. If the child speaks on this occasion, it is likely that the first speaker will interrupt him. This in turn will result in the child's silence, since his partner's voice has become an occasion for his silence. If this happens frequently enough, repetitions and long pauses may become a recurring pattern in the child's speech. The child must determine when a silence in his conversational partner is merely a pause and when it is actually a signal for him to speak (without interruption). If the speech patterns of the partner are persistently of the sort described, the child may emit the first sound and wait briefly for the interruption. If the interruption is not forthcoming he repeats the first sound as part of the originally intended message unit and continues with the remainder of his utterances. The repetition response may be maintained in great strength under such circumstances.

Case histories of families and clinical observations reveal many other specific occasions for dysfluency in the child's speech involving aversive stimulation and states of deprivation in the child's environment. These include maintaining too high a level of excitement and activity; requiring too fast a pace of verbal and nonverbal activity in the family; pressuring the child for answers to questions; unconsciously arranging situations that are consistently frustrating for the child; employing inconsistent and sometimes confusing disciplinary and child-rearing practices; permitting the occurrence of highly charged emotional interactions between parents in front of the child; consciously or unconsciously allowing the teasing or frightening of the child; lack of parental attention; and changing environments, in families who move a great deal.

In summary, it has been suggested that dysfluency may occur as a normal speech reaction to abnormal environmental events. Professional intervention may be required to develop strategies for the modification of the environment. Such environmental manipulation has had a high rate of success in reducing speech dysfluencies in young children. Aversive stimulation, states of deprivation, and competition for talking time could be potent factors in such situations. There appear to be some children who have a reduced tolerance for even the usually encountered pressures of everyday living. Under such circumstances, both environmental modification and direct desensitization therapy with the child may be in order to develop greater tolerance for normally encountered pressures in the home.

STUTTERING

There is no reason to believe, once stuttering has been diagnosed, that the young stutterer is immune from the contingencies and controls suggested as operating in normal dysfluency as a reaction to environmental pressure. In fact, it appears that not only do these contingencies continue when and if stuttering develops, but they may contribute to the more complicated forms and circumstances of dysfluency that have come to be known as stuttering. However, it should be recognized that stuttering consists of much more than what the stutterer makes available for public observation. There seems to be a private side to stuttering that the stutterer makes public only occasionally. Of course, if a clinician expects to do more than manipulate his preconceived ideas of this private side of stuttering, he has to help the stutterer make these hidden factors available for examination, analysis, and therapeutic manipulation.

There appear to be three important processes that differentiate stuttering from normal dysfluency and from dysfluency related to environmental pressures. First, the form of the dysfluency may have undergone some deterioration or change, so that it now may be characterized by muscular tension and forcing. Second, there is a greater consistency in the loci of stuttering. Bloodstein (1960) has suggested that stutterers are consistently dysfluent on the same words, while nonstutterers are not. It should be pointed out, however, that consistency of loci is only one form of consistency, and it may well be the only form that differentiates stutterers from nonstutterers. There is also consistency in the form of the dysfluency (repetition, pause, prolongation), in the rate of emission of dysfluency, and in the grammatical forms in which dysfluency occurs. These types of consistencies of dysfluencies may not differentiate stutterers from nonstutterers, and it is the specific consistency of loci that has such diagnostic significance (McCann, 1967).

Third, the dysfluency may no longer be simply a response to an abnormal amount of environmental pressure, but it may also be the occasion for public and private evaluative verbal responses by the stutterer. This behavioral view of the dynamics of stuttering derives in part from the semantogenic point of view of stuttering developed by Johnson and his students (Johnson, 1958). However, it is suggested that the dysfluencies of the stutterer are under the control of their consequent events, some of which emanate from the stutterer's environment through listeners and some of which emanate from the stutterer himself as he hears, monitors, reacts to, and changes his speech responses. The stutterer may rehearse, try to avoid talking, try to keep talking, try to avoid silent pauses, try to change aversive forms of speech responses, try to avoid the dysfluency, try to avoid listeners' reactions, engage in ritualistic motor and verbal behavior he believes helps him to talk (eye blinking, foot tapping, repeated interjections), and try to avoid his aversive evaluations of helplessness and being victimized. He may vacillate from one response to the other. Often internal and external cues become evoking stimuli for stuttering and allied verbal and motor responses. Among such cues are fleeting sensations of muscular movement during speech articulation, situational events like group discussions, particular people, and objects like telephones. Stutterers also report that specific sounds or words evoke their stuttering responses.

Although stuttering may have many painful consequences for the stutterer, such behavior may also provide some payoffs for him. Case histories and observation consistently reveal that the stutterer obtains special privileges, holds a listener's attention, forces a polite listener's silence during his struggle behavior, and develops a handy excuse for difficulties and failures quite unrelated to stuttering. From this brief overview of stuttering, it should be obvious that this can be an extremely complicated behavioral problem. Some of the problem is public, while some of it is private. Some of the problem can be identified at a purely motor level in terms of the specific forms of the speech response, while other aspects of the problem can be identified by the language content and themes revealed in the stutterer's overt speech utterances. One hypothesis offered about stuttering is that there appears to be some relation between the way a stutterer thinks and feels about himself and his speech (self-generated consequence of stuttering) as reflected in what he overtly says to a clinician, and the dysfluent motor aspects of his speech known as stuttering. The task for the clinician is to identify those variables both within and outside the stutterer that exercise control over his stuttering.

For very young children who are reacting to environmental pressure by emitting speech dysfluencies (neither normal dysfluency nor stuttering), the prognosis traditionally has been quite favorable. The goals of professional intervention (indirect environmental manipulation) in this situation have been speech that would not be differentiated as abnormal. However, the circumstances for such speech dysfluency should not be permitted to persist with the hopes that the child will outgrow the problem. The child will not outgrow persistent, continued abnormal environmental pressure. The problem is not within the child, but rather in his environment and it is, therefore, his environment that should receive appropriate professional attention. Interestingly, it is with this type of problem that speech pathologists have enjoyed their highest rate of success.

For the problem of stuttering in children and adults, the prognosis has been much less favorable and the goals and results of therapy more variable. In general, it appears that the younger the stutterer, the more favorable the prognosis. However, there is a period of psychosocial development, both just before and just after puberty, during which clinicians and their stutterers have experienced much frustration and mixed degrees of success.

SUMMARY

Any discussion of the development of stuttering must necessarily include a consideration of other clinical entities with which stuttering is sometimes confused and from which it must be differentiated. It is suggested that the diagnostician must differentiate among normal dysfluency, dysfluency associated with environmental pressure, and stuttering. This diagnostic evaluation is based in part on a consideration of the topography of the child's speech responses and the circumstances prevailing when these responses occur. It is specifically suggested that dysfluency and stuttering responses, as well as those events that seem to evoke these responses, are under the control of the consequences generated by such speech responses. In therapy, the clinician has the task of modifying those variables operating in the speaker's environment as well as those reactions emanating from the stutterer that influence the appearance of dysfluency and stuttering.

4

....

Some
General Considerations
of Therapy

WHAT TO CHANGE
AND HOW TO CHANGE IT

The common factor in all therapy is *change,* whether it be change in the individual's perception, attitude, behavior, or environment. By definition, clinicians are in the business of forcing, facilitating, or observing change. The primary questions for the clinician are, "What should I attempt to change in therapy?" and "How should I attempt to bring about this change?" The answers to these two questions ultimately embrace all the principles that underlie therapeutic transactions.

The question of what to change involves the establishment of behavioral goals and subgoals and the designation of specific responses and events that are targeted for change. The decisions about goals and target responses are derived from our view of the problem. They imply a point of view on our part of what constitutes an optimum form or range of behaviors and circumstances for an individual stutterer. For example, the decision may be to modify the speech of the stutterer, or to change his self-perception, or to change the evaluative behaviors of his parents, or to reorganize the occasions for speaking encounters in the home. Each of these possibilities as end goals should derive from a set of events that may emerge during our evaluations as pertinent factors in the problem. To change such events means that we have decided that the current state of affairs relative to these events is not optimal and that we have some notion of what is optimal. It is this conception of "optimal" behavior and circumstances that is viewed as our ultimate goal. Our views of what constitutes an optimal circumstance for an individual come from many sources. We are really talking about a much larger problem for clinicians and theorists alike in that we are dealing with the issue of defining what constitutes appropriate speech, good mental health, individual happiness, and social adjustment. Our society and culture provide rules for accepting and tolerating a broad range of behaviors and events by members of a community. Our cultural value system also provides boundaries and constraints on individuals. Family and religious value systems also contribute to the concepts we employ regarding optimal conditions for living in various group arrangements. Our own personal histories and theories help us to decide on ultimate end goals for therapy.

From a behavioral standpoint we might try to think about these things in terms of individual behaviors that will generate from society positive reinforcers for the stutterer. Although this may seem simplistic, it can sometimes get complex. For example, fluency will probably generate approval from a mother. But will greater talkativeness generate acceptance from a sibling? There may be times when collisions occur; for example, increased assertiveness and independence by a young child can upset the usual system of interaction in the home, and therefore generate penalties for the child. In instances like these a judgment has to be made about the value (long- and short-term) of the new behavior for generating positive reinforcers over the entire range of the child's system of living. If a restricted circumstance generates penalty, then it should be analyzed and perhaps modified, but should not necessarily become the sole reason for making a decision about the value of a particular end goal behavior.

The question of how to bring about the change is a question of process and tactics. There are a number of procedural issues to be considered. Decisions have to be made about how we provide *occasions* for the stutterer to emit his target behavior. A *system for evaluating progress* has to be established. We have to decide on the *form and type of contingent consequences* we are going to employ and the *schedules* on which we will provide these consequences. We have to decide on the format to be employed. This would include such issues as whether we are going to *shape* the stutterer's behavior from some starting point of his own, or whether we are going to give the stutterer *verbal instructions* to behave in a certain way, or whether we are going to provide a *model for the stutterer to match.* Finally, decisions about carryover and making the stutterer responsible for himself have to be translated into clinical tactics and transactions. Some of these decisions must be made before therapy begins, while others may be made afterwards.

For the stutterer's listeners, for most clinicians, and, ostensibly, for the stutterer, what most prominently needs change is the fluency pattern. Having a stutterer become fluent is a goal that, with one addition, is a goal of therapy we would endorse. That addition is adverbial and the word is *comfortably.* Newly and finally stated the goal of therapy is to produce a speaker who is comfortably fluent. This speaker will speak fluently without rehearsal or anticipation, without consciously monitoring his fluency pattern, and with the normal fluency disruptions of most people. To quote one of our own clients, the stutterer successful in therapy will just "open up my mouth and talk like everybody else whenever and wherever I want to."

In pursuing this goal, most frustrating, perhaps, is the fact that almost any method for the amelioration of stuttering has succeeded at least once. Anecdotes of such successes have existed since Demosthenes and their echoes reverberate in clinics even to this day.

Most professional methods of treatment have also ameliorated stuttering for varying periods of time. Because stuttering has been reduced or eliminated by a variety of procedures, it would seem reasonable to postulate that different techniques have differences that are only superficial, and that underlying these differences are some common components or processes. Armchair guesses about the common components include: someone cares; something is being done; strong faith in the therapy or clinician by the stutterer; or I'm (the stutterer) doing something.

Just as many therapeutic methods have succeeded at least once, so have many of these same methods failed, in most cases, repeatedly. The record is not an encouraging one, because failures exceed successes, particularly when the problem of carryover is considered. Carryover, the extension of therapeutic successes outside of therapy and beyond therapy in time, is the sandbar that has grounded many a method once heralded and acclaimed. This would seem to indicate that either therapeutic procedures have been inadequate or were terminated prematurely.

The fact that no one clinical procedure for the amelioration of stuttering can at present be said to be superior to any other would seem to indicate that method-comparison studies are not the most fruitful, particularly if only the outcomes of the respective methods are compared. What seems more important is to examine the *process* of therapy regardless of the label applied to the method of therapy. Therefore, instead of saying categorically what method was used, one describes what actually occurred in the moment-to-moment progression of therapy.

Such an approach is compatible with the operant approach this book advocates for structuring stuttering therapy. It is advocated for a number of reasons, three of which are prominent here. First, it relies heavily upon the description of behaviors of both client and clinician. An operant clinician must describe exactly what he did, what the client did in consequence, what he did in consequence, and so on. If he does not do this, the operant clinician is apparently just exploiting the term "operant" for his own purposes. Second, the operant approach does not assign *a priori* hierarchical values to stuttering behaviors. Fewer assumptions are made about stuttering in general, or about a client and his stuttering in particular. Third is that the operant method can be used as a meta-method. *It can be used as a method to describe other methods.* For example, suppose Clinician A reports that he is using the indirect method in therapy while Clinician B reports using a direct method. Using the operant method as a meta-method, we would observe both clinicians at work and describe the time-sequenced behaviors that occurred. We could label descriptions Method A or Method B but it would not be necessary to do so. To reduce various therapeutic approaches to the behavioral dimension places them on a common scale, permitting the detection of overlapping therapeutic processes as well as manifest differences. This reduction is possible when one uses the operant method as a meta-method.

The use of the meta-method approach does not necessarily denigrate the contribution of a particular theory. The fact that a clinician, who is using method A, can have his therapeutic behaviors comprehensively described in operant terminology testifies only to the ability of operant analyses to describe the processes of therapy or the implementation of therapy. The plan or design of therapy is best suggested by existing theoretical, experimental, or empirical formulations, and in this sense, the value of these formulations survive.

To amplify these points, an exercise we often use in introductory Problems of Speech classes will be presented. Before lecturing to the class on theories of stuttering we often ask members of the class to list things stutterers do that we can see or hear; things stutterers say they do; things we infer; and things stutterers infer. For convenience we place the observational characteristics under the category labeled "Overt" and the inferential characteristics in the category "Covert." A typical result of this exercise would be as follows:

Overt: Repeats words, syllables, phrases; blocks on words; moves arms and legs; closes eyes; has jerky head movements; looks away; uses stereotyped phrases like "you know" and "ah well"; holds breath when talking; usually all right when he gets started; grinds teeth.

Covert: Is nervous; is anxious; is afraid; is hostile; changes words; says "I don't know" when he knows; avoids talking situations; holds back feelings; holds back telling the truth.

Parenthetically, it is interesting to note the power of a label. Students asked to enumerate a stutterer's characteristics typically give lengthy lists but seldom mention fluent speech as a characteristic, whereas in fact, all stutterers are fluent at times and most stutterers utter more fluent words than dysfluent ones.

At any rate, the importance of a list like the one above is that it demonstrates the large number of behaviors that can be directly or indirectly manipulated in therapy. In designing a program many options are available and in this sense an operant approach is not restrictive.

In terms of theoretical, experimental, or empirical orientations it can be seen that the list includes those behaviors or attributes that many theorists would deem critical to the acquisition and/or maintenance of stuttering. Thus, an operant program utilizing these characteristics is compatible with many theoretical approaches in that it is capable of incorporating a number of theoretical directives. At the same time a program is not bound by these directives.

When a clinician plans his therapy, including his instructions to the client and the responses that he will make to the client's responses, a therapy program emerges. A therapy program, then, is a set of prescribed clinician responses to be made in contingent response to the client's responses. At first glance this definition of a therapy program may seem severely restrictive. It is, in the sense that once the program is established the clinician's behavior is determined. However, in the establishment or design phase there are extensive opportunities for creative experimentation.

As an exercise we will now construct two therapy programs to illustrate some pertinent issues in employing operant-based therapy. Table 4.1 illustrates such an arrangement.

Reading through this program, a not unsurprising first reaction is "how boring and repetitious." This is characteristic of programs with specific clinical instructions. What must be remembered is that the program was not designed to stimulate the reader but to bring about fluency in stutterers for whom it was designed. Of course, we could have reduced the amount of space used for presenting the program by ditto marks, subscripts, and so on, and normally we would have, but here we intended to create an awareness of the repetition inherent in programs.

The tedium experienced in reading the program is often experienced in executing the program. It should be apparent that if this particular program were adopted we would forfeit our freedom to respond to the

TABLE 4.1. Sample Sentence Fluency Reinforcement Therapy Program.

Step	Instruction
Begin here	Go to Step 1.
1	Recite single words simultaneously with the stutterer. When 5 in sequence are said fluently go to Step 2.
2	Ask the stutterer to think of any word he can say fluently and to say it. Repeat this request 4 times. If each of the 5 words is said fluently, say, "Very good," and move to Step 3; if not, return to Step 1.
3	Ask the stutterer to think of any 2 words he can say fluently and to say them. Repeat this request 4 times. If each of the pairs is said fluently, say, "Very good," and move to Step 4; if not, return to Step 2.
4	Ask the stutterer to think of any 3 words he can say fluently and to say them. Repeat this request 4 times. If each of the word triplets is said fluently, say, "Very good," and move to Step 5; if not, return to Step 3.
5	Ask the stutterer to think of any 4 words he can say fluently and to say them. Repeat the request 4 times. If each of the 4-word sets is said fluently, say, "Very good," and move to Step 6; if not, return to Step 4.
6	Ask the stutterer to think of any 5 words he can say fluently and to say them. Repeat the request 4 times. If each of the 5-word sets is said fluently, say, "Very good," and move to Step 7; if not, return to Step 5.
7	Ask the stutterer to think of a sentence he can say fluently and to say it. Repeat the request 4 times. If each sentence is said fluently, say, "Very good," and move to Step 8; if not, return to Step 6.
8	Ask the stutterer to speak fluently for 1 minute. If he stutters more than once, return to Step 7; otherwise, say, "Very good," and move to Step 9.
9	Ask the stutterer to speak fluently for 5 minutes. If he stutters more than 5 times, return to Step 8; otherwise, say, "Very good," and move to Step 10.
10	Ask the stutterer to speak fluently for 10 minutes. If he stutters more than 10 times, return to Step 9; otherwise, say, "Very good," and move to Step 11.
11	Ask the stutterer to speak fluently for 20 minutes. If he stutters more than 20 times, return to Step 10; otherwise, say, "Very good," and move to Step 12.
12	Ask the stutterer to speak fluently for 40 minutes. If he stutters more than 40 times, return to Step 11; otherwise, say, "Very good," and move to Step 13.
13	Ask the stutterer to choose 3 outside situations when you can observe his speech. If he stutters on more than 1 percent of his words in any of the situations, return to Step 12; otherwise, discharge the stutterer from therapy with your best wishes.

content of our stutterer's speech and to our own impulses. We would be "automated," our responses predetermined. All decisions for the entire therapy experience from entry to discharge are contained in the program and are not a function of the clinician's judgment. Many times it seems that negative reactions to the development and application of therapeutic programs are ostensibly directed at their lack of validity, whereas part of these reactions may be due to this programming or automating of the clinician. Elaborate, highly symbolic, and abstract interpretations and

TABLE 4.2.   Sample Flash Card Fluency Reinforcement Program.

Type Trial	Instructions to Client	Clinician's Contingent Response
1 Baseline	Read the sentence on the card	None
2 Conditioning	Same	React to each fluent response with "Good job"
3 Conditioning	Same	Same
4 Conditioning	Same	Same
5 Conditioning	Same	Same

reflections may stimulate us intellectually but may not necessarily be the most efficacious approach to therapy.

Our second illustrative program has two steps: baseline and conditioning. The response to be conditioned or learned is the production of fluent sentences. For this program we have 100 flash cards upon which are printed sentences, one per card. During the baseline period we have the stutterer read the cards in sequence and note the number of sentences where an incident of stuttering has occurred. This is our baseline measure. In preparation for the conditioning period of our program we decide upon the response to be conditioned, the type of contingent response to use, and the means of dispensing it. The information collected in the baseline in part determines the response (s) to be conditioned. In our example, we note the number of flash card sentences where an episode of stuttering occurs. By simple subtraction we also have the number of "fluent" cards, i.e., the number of sentences read without stuttering. We therefore have available baseline data on both stuttering and fluency. We decide to focus on fluent responses and we operationally define a fluent response as fluent reading of a sentence presented on a flash card. Each time the stutterer exhibits a fluent response we decide to react contingently with a verbal response, "Good job." We withhold this response when a stuttering response is exhibited; namely, when one or more occurrences of stuttering are exhibited in reading a sentence from the flash card. However, we could just as easily decide to consequate stuttered sentences with disapproval by the clinician. With these decisions made we begin the first conditioning session. We have the stutterer read the cards and we react contingently according to the precepts of the therapy program we established. Schematically we could represent our therapy program at this point in Table 4.2. Let us now supply some numbers to serve as hypothetical results in the application of our program. Let them be as follows:

*Number of Fluent Responses
per 100 Cards*

Baseline Period	67
Conditioning Trial 1	71
Conditioning Trial 2	77
Conditioning Trial 3	83
Conditioning Trial 4	89
Conditioning Trial 5	91

From a clinician's point of view the data generated by the program appear encouraging. An increased number of fluent sentences were emitted with each successive conditioning trial. To continue with the conditioning trials one would assume that more fluent sentences would be emitted until the upper limit of 100 fluent sentences were obtained.

If we were to evaluate our program at this point we could ask a countless number of questions. Some prominent ones would include:

1. Have we conditioned our stutterer—has he learned to be fluent?
2. Will the fluency acquired while reading cards generalize to conversational situations inside and outside the clinic?
3. What would we have done if the therapy program failed to give the results desired?

In response to question one, we cannot be sure that our stutterer has increased his fluency as a result of the program. Since our stutterer was asked to read the same 100 cards during each session, the increase in fluency may be a product of adaptation. Adaptation is the progressive decrease in the frequency of stuttering on repeated readings of the same material. To control for adaptation we could have a large pool of cards, say 1,000 instead of 100, and we could randomize their presentation. Another possibility that would contraindicate conditioning or learning fluency would be that our baseline measure was inadequate. Assuming that we controlled for adaptation, there remains the possibility that the same or similar results could have occurred in the absence of any clinician contingent responding or in the absence of any conditioning sessions. In other words, if we would have run six baseline trials we might have observed a systematic decrease in the number of stuttering responses. This possibility suggests that we should acquire an adequate baseline measure. A criterion for an adequate baseline is that you observe the behavior until there are no longer any systematic changes in the behavior over time, increases or decreases. Variations are possible but they should appear random and not systematic. Suppose in our program we conducted five baseline trials and obtained 65, 69, 63, 71, and 67 fluent responses. Because there appears to be a random variation of fluent responses around the average of 67 we can conclude that we have an adequate baseline and can proceed with the conditioning trials in an attempt to increase the number of fluent responses.

A final test to determine whether or not conditioning has occurred is to have the clinician withhold his contingent response, "Good job," after each fluent response. When this is done after conditioning trials the process is called *extinction*. In extinction we repeat the conditions of baseline after conditioning. If the clinician's contingent responding is indeed instrumental in evoking more fluent responses then the withdrawal of contingent responses should lead to a reinstatement of more stuttered responses. The extinction process poses a number of problems for clinicians, the most prominent being that of reinstating an undesirable behavior such as stuttering. It is here that the clinician and the experimentalist disagree. The clinician is interested in assisting the stutterer in becoming comfortably fluent while the experimentalist is interested in studying the effects of an essentially infinite number of variables on stuttering and fluency. There is no simple solution to this problem. The tendency among clinicians using operant procedures is to use extinction minimally particularly if it means the possible reinstatement of stuttering.

A second but related problem posed by extinction relates to the generalization of fluency. If a stutterer becomes fluent under our program we infer that it is a result of conditioning or the clinician's contingent responding. Therefore, when the stutterer is not reading the cards, when he is talking inside and outside of therapy, we have in a sense an extinction situation since listeners are not responding contingently to his fluent responses. The essence of this dilemma is that we cannot, by definition, expect any carryover outside of an operant therapy program that has not been included in that program. It is true that we could extend our program to cover a large number of speaking situations and provide contingent responses in these situations. But we cannot condition the stutterer throughout life. At some point we want him to be comfortably fluent and independent of us and our contingencies. This may require that the stutterer experience perceptual changes as well as motor changes in his speech.

In answer to question two, we do not know if the fluency acquired in the pilot therapy program would generalize to other speaking situations. We do know that it was not part of that phase of the program.

Question three asks if the program can accommodate failure. The term failure has a common meaning, that the stutterer is not becoming fluent; and a technical meaning, that the clinician's contingent response, "Good job," is not a positive reinforcer. The number of fluent responses the stutterer exhibited in the conditioning sessions did not systematically increase from the baseline frequency. There are a number of procedures in program design for assisting the stutterer who is unsuccessful in becoming fluent. At the extremes, of course, we have either program abandonment or continued conditioning trials. Between these extremes is usually a program so comprehensive in terms of the number of conditioning steps that the stutterer begins at a level where he experiences success and then moves to the next step in the program. Movement to any new step in the program is contingent upon success in the previous step. If there is failure in any advanced step the stutterer returns to a previous step in the program. The basic notion underlying this movement in a program is that the acquisition of conversational fluency proceeds gradually, as does the acquisition of other motoric behaviors. Thus a therapy program designed to evoke fluency must take into account the typical learning curve of gradual acquisition. If a clinician tests a therapeutic program and finds that one step of the program is particularly difficult, that is, the stutterer does not systematically depart in the desired direction from baseline, he must break the difficult step into a number of smaller steps.

We began this section by presenting the general issues and decisions we have to make about the processes and content of therapy. We also presented two hypothetical therapy programs and defined the necessary operational concepts as we progressed. The purpose was to introduce some rudimentary considerations in therapeutic program construction. The boredom of the fluency word program and the fragmentary nature of the flash card program make them easy targets for criticism. It is most important to note that the criticisms we were able to direct at the flash card program were in part due to the detailed description given of the program. In designing a therapy program we comprehensively describe the operations of the program. This openness makes evaluation and criticism easier. Therefore, as we design and apply our therapeutic programs we should be prepared for criticism of our efforts made possible by our own detailed description of our therapeutic strategies. It is this same description that permits each of us to be a critic of his own work. Reasoned revision and modifications can be made in our programs on the basis of the records of previous attempts.

DEFINING
THE TARGET RESPONSE

By now it should have become increasingly evident that the basic operant paradigm, $S \rightarrow R \rightarrow Rf$, is an essentially content-free form. When using this model in a therapy situation we commit ourselves to a particular form of observing and responding. We do not, however, commit ourselves necessarily to observing and contingently responding to any designated response. We can compare the basic paradigm to an algebraic equation in that the equation is an expression without content; it only acquires meaning in application. Thus, we can let the X of an equation be the length of a room, the circumference of a circle, or whatever we choose. In like manner, the R in the basic paradigm can be an arm movement, an overt stuttering episode, or a statement of self-denigration. While we do not randomly choose responses to condition in therapy, we must remember that the model does not restrict the responses to which we can react contingently. Moreover, it does not determine the specific kind of contingent response we will make. A more detailed discussion of our choice behavior will follow below.

When we choose to react contingently to a response such as a stuttering episode, and we do this repeatedly, we will find upon close observation that the stuttering responses are not identical. There is a group of responses that resemble each other and we call any member of that group a stuttering response. This is similar to the linguistic concept of a phoneme, where there are many variations of a particular sound of the language within and across speakers. These variations are essentially ignored and members of the linguistic community perceive the family of sounds, technically called allophones, as one sound. In operant conditioning the family of responses is called an *operant*. Technically, then, when we say we are conditioning a response we are in reality conditioning, with repeated trials, an operant (a class of equivalent responses), thus the term *operant conditioning*.

The importance of this discussion of individual responses and operants (classes of individual responses) relates to response definition. When defining an operant we must decide the number and the degree of variations we are willing to include in this response family or group. We readily think of repetitions, prolongations, and blocks, seemingly the most universal overt characteristics of stuttering, but there also are many behavioral and cognitive postures and sets that precede, accompany, or immediately follow stuttering episodes. These peripheral components seem more individual and less universal as they vary more from stutterer to stutterer. The question is whether or not the peripheral components should be included in our definition of the stuttering operant. The observational test for answering the question is the test of co-occurrence. Those behaviors and attitudes that co-occur, either sequentially or simultaneously, with the act of stuttering should most probably be included in the definition of the stuttering operant. The behavioral test for answering the question consists of manipulating, by conditioning methods, one component or response of the operant. If the definition of the operant for a particular stutterer is valid then we should observe changes in the frequency of occurrence of all responses included in the definition of the operant. A clinical example of this validation process concerns an adult female stutterer who consistently protruded her tongue before exhibiting stuttering episodes. Thus there was co-occurrence (tongue protrusion and stuttering). We began a mild verbal punishment program for the tongue protrusion saying "tongue," or something similar each time she protruded her tongue. With this strategy in effect not only did we see a reduction in tongue protrusion but in stuttering as well, which leads us to believe that tongue protrusion responses were members of the stuttering operant. Results in this case and in many others showed that verbal output was not suppressed, in other words, that it is possible to isolate stuttering responses from speaking responses in general. However, the same responses that constitute an operant for one stutterer may not function similarly for another stutterer.

Further difficulties related to the definition of the operant "stuttering" can be seen when we consider the various terms used to describe the behavior. Two of these terms are sufficient to account for the dilemma. They are *stuttering* and *dysfluency*. The nomenclature suggests only stutterers are capable of stuttering while both stutterers and nonstutterers are capable of exhibiting dysfluencies. Therefore, if we are conditioning the operant "dysfluency," we will be contingently reacting to many behaviors exhibited by nonstutterers. If it is our specific goal to suppress dysfluent responses we will be setting a goal for our stutterer that is not reached by nonstutterers, since the speech of nonstutterers is peppered with dysfluencies. We prefer the term "stuttering" to the more general term "dysfluency." This preference has no esthetic basis but reflects our concerns with validity. Although the difference between the terms is qualitative, there are some discernible characteristics between stuttering and dysfluency. The nonstuttering dysfluent person will usually not display single sound or syllable repetitions or tonic and clonic blocks; his dysfluencies will usually be restricted to the larger linguistic units, whole words and phrases. The nonstutterer will not react to his dysfluencies in the same way that the stutterer will. Both the stutterer and nonstutterer may exhibit the same dysfluency but their resultant reactions will differ.

Even with these distinctions in mind there is still an area of uncertainty between stuttering and normal dysfluency. This area of uncertainty takes on significant importance when we consider the diagnosis of children, particularly with reference to Johnson's semantogenic theory (Johnson, 1958), where the application of the label "stuttering" to normal dysfluencies may indeed be responsible for the child developing into a full-blown stutterer. With adult stutterers, too, we believe that a distinction should be made between dysfluency and stuttering. Though there is a possible overlap between the two classes of behavior, we should still attempt to distinguish between them. Otherwise we may be penalizing the stutterer for emitting essentially normal behavior. Some procedures for defining the operant "stuttering" are to establish reliability with oneself, establish reliability with other clinicians, and establish reliability with the stutterer. In establishing self-reliability we make repeated judgments on the same sample of speech by the stutterer. A video and/or audio recording is, of course, necessary. We can compare our judgments by using percentages or correlation coefficients. The former is an absolute measure of agreement while the latter shows relative agreement. When establishing reliability with another clinician or with the stutterer, we compare our judgments with the respective participant.

In the process of establishing reliability of judgment, questions of validity will necessarily emerge. By a valid judgment we mean that what we have judged to be stuttering is indeed stuttering. Of course, we have no definitive test to determine the occurrence of stuttering. But we should not be discouraged, because any time we attempt to establish reliability we are forced to examine our criteria for labeling certain behaviors as unique to stuttering. These criteria in turn become our definition of stuttering. We believe it is helpful in many cases to establish reliability with the stutterer. In the process we can validate our own judgment against the stutterer's judgment. While we do not recommend wholesale adoption of the stutterer's criteria, some reliance should be placed on his judgment, since he has access to more information about his behaviors on the sensory and perceptual level. Operationally we have found that where both stutterer and clinician agree that an exhibited behavior was stuttering, we have reasonable assurance that a valid judgment was made. And, when the percentage of agreement is of high magnitude, such assurance is correspondingly enhanced. These parallel judgments, of course, must be made independently.

THE EVOKING STIMULUS

So far in our discussion of the operant paradigm we have said little about the evoking stimulus except that it is difficult to identify. We simply do not know the event or events that trigger a specific stuttering episode. We can, as many have, speculate about the specific triggering mechanisms for stuttering. They range from the isolated identifiable stimuli to hypothetical constructs. Thus we can speculate that stuttering is triggered by a particular linguistic unit in a word, say an initial phoneme, or by some construct such as fear or anxiety. Stutterers are capable of listing a variety of evoking stimuli for stuttering and often contradict themselves in doing so. It is not unusual for a stutterer to report, "I just can't say the 's' words," and contradict himself by saying, "say" fluently.

In our observations the most reliable stimulus configuration is situational and/or interpersonal. We have seen stutterers who stuttered only when they were in a particular setting. It was as though this setting were the stimulus for their stuttering while other settings evoked fluency. In like manner stuttering seems to be evoked in the presence of certain individuals, such as parents or teachers. We have had clients who became fluent outside of therapy but not inside; others were just the opposite. It was as though the therapy room was the stimulus for fluency since they stuttered in almost all other situations. Interpersonally we have seen stutterers who seemed to be controlled by the presence of specific individuals. Their presence seemed to be the occasion for the stutterer to stutter. One such stutterer was essentially fluent except with an old shopkeeper from whom he made purchases as a child. The shopkeeper was the last vestige stimulus for the man's stuttering.

Although situational and interpersonal variables can reliably evoke fluency or stuttering, the variables are nonetheless highly individualized. This is, of course, not unexpected since each stutterer brings to therapy a unique history. The individual nature of these stimulus control variables, however, poses a problem for the clinician interested in developing therapy programs with general applicability. We strive to develop programs that can ameliorate stuttering in the majority of stutterers, but at present we modify these programs to accommodate for individual differences among stutterers. We could, perhaps, develop a program so comprehensive that it would contain almost every conceivable modification. Such a program would perhaps be unmanageable because of the large number of steps and stages required.

The S^D (discriminative stimulus) is an important component of the question being discussed. During clinical interviews, the S^D may be elusive and time-consuming to establish. Quite often it is the most neglected aspect of the operant paradigm. When we ask a stutterer to read a flash card, a discriminative stimulus is given, and under normal circumstances the stutterer will read the card and not look at his watch and tell us what time it is. When one stimulus reliably evokes one of many possible responses, the stimulus is said to be a discriminative stimulus. In the pilot flash card program discussed earlier the clinician contingently responded with, "Good job," when the stutterer read a card fluently. We can regard the stutterer's fluent response as the discriminative stimulus for the clinician's "Good job" response. Thus in therapy, through the course of clinician-client interchanges, we have a cascade of stimuli and responses. When the statement of one participant directs or determines the behavior of the second, we can say that the utterance of the first is the discriminative stimulus for the response of the second, which in turn can serve as the discriminative stimulus for the first participant's second response and so on. However, when we consider these respective verbal responses as discriminative stimuli that evoke specific responses, we must recognize the limitations. We can say, "Read a card," to a stutterer, and there is a high probability that he will read the card if it is available. However, if we say, "Speak fluently for an hour," we may see less compliance. The stutterer may not be fluent for an hour; in fact, he may stutter within the first minute. The gist of this discussion is that stimuli are discriminative when they can predictably evoke a designated response. To the extent that people answer questions when asked or engage in interactions according to the social rules of graciousness implies that a response from one is a stimulus for the second. It is only a discriminative stimulus in the sense that a response from one evokes a response from the other, the simple give-and-take of conversation. For example, if when asked a series of 50 questions a stutterer answers, but stutters during only 25 of his answers, we might infer that "questions" are a discriminative stimulus for "answers," but not necessarily for "stuttered answers." To label a verbal statement a discriminative stimulus is inaccurate if the occurrence of that stimulus fails to evoke reliably a designated response.

It is probably true that certain stimulus configurations take on controlling properties during the course of therapy. For example, the stutterer who acquires fluency in the clinic is probably under control of the clinic environment and the people therein. Placed in this environment there is a high probability that he will be fluent. At times conversational themes seem to evoke fluency. We have had stutterers who predictably would become fluent when they talked about the subject of stuttering.

It is because of these problems associated with the evoking stimulus that we focus most intensely upon the stutterer's operant responses. We can more reliably identify the responses and react to them contingently than can we identify stimuli that will evoke fluency or stuttering.

The problem for the clinician is that there may be a number of stimuli, many of which are not under his control, that can evoke stuttering during a therapy session. Our interest in the evoking stimulus is that our ability to change the stutterer's responses may depend on our ability to control not only the consequences of responses, but also the occasions for their emission.

The clinician is in a position to try to establish such control and bring about the desirable changes by arranging for the occurrence of certain consequences in the presence of certain stimuli. These stimuli gain their evocative powers by being temporally bound to the consequent event.

The importance of the degree of stimulus control by the clinician is not totally understood and may vary with the particular therapy program employed. For example, in a delayed auditory feedback (DAF) therapy program, the stutterer hears his own voice at a slight delay, measured in milliseconds. This delay is disruptive and aversive but its effect can be lessened by slowing down one's speech. The presentation of this aversive stimulus (delayed auditory feedback) is shared by the stutterer and the clinician. The clinician makes available the equipment, but the stutterer must talk to create the aversive delayed feedback. The response by the stutterer of prolonged and slower speech has the consequence of lessening the disruptive effects of delay.

In programs designed to modify the forms of stuttering, the occasion for "modification" behavior is almost completely under the stimulus control of the stutterer, since it depends on the occurrence of stuttering responses by the stutterer. Stuttering cannot be modified if the stutterer doesn't stutter.

This problem of the evoking stimulus for stuttering or fluency highlights the dyadic nature of therapy. The clinician depends on the stutterer to emit responses over which he may exercise little stimulus control. The stutterer depends on the clinician to provide consequences for his responses that will affect their occurrence in therapeutic and desirable ways.

THE CONTINGENT CONSEQUENCE

Some people have characterized therapy as the search by the clinician for an effective reinforcer, a search for some type of event that we can provide as a contingent consequence. Although we may not be able to arrange easily for the occurrence of evoking stimuli, and we may have to wait for the stutterer to emit certain target responses, we are in a good position to provide significant contingent consequences for the stutterer's behavior. We should recognize that we may better be able to provide consequences than to deal with either of the earlier occurring elements of the conditioning paradigm ($S^D \rightarrow R$). We should also recognize that it is in this element of the paradigm, the reinforcing event (Rf), that the power of the law of effect resides (Thorndike, 1933). It is the contingent consequence that gives the S^D its evocatory properties. And it is the contingent consequence that affects the probability of occurrence of the target response of the stutterer. S^D's do not exist without Rf's. However, as awesome and powerful and privileged as the clinician's position and functioning as a contingent consequator might appear, even here, it is a shared responsibility. In all likelihood there are a number of consequences exercising control over the stutterer's responses. The clinician may see a stutterer in therapy from one to three or four hours a week out of a total of approximately 112 hours a week the stutterer may be socially active. Ninety-seven percent of the time the stutterer is exposed to other people, to other events, and to other stimuli, many of which may exercise control over his responses and may or may not be congruent with the clinician's transactions.

The choice of the type of contingent consequence we employ in therapy is dictated by the target response emitted by the stutterer we elect to deal with. In general, we try to reduce the frequency of undesirable responses and increase the frequency of desirable responses. We positively reinforce fluency to increase it or we highlight or aversively stimulate stuttering to reduce it. We may give approval, acceptance, and understanding of statements that reflect the stutterer's insight, in an effort to increase their frequency, and give disapproval and rejection of statements that reflect the stutterer's feelings of helplessness, victimization, and lack of self-responsibility, in an effort to reduce their frequency. The forms that these contingent events take need vary only with the constraints of their relative effectiveness, viability, and availability. Positive reinforcers have ranged from candy, money, toys, points, and tokens to approval, acceptance, understanding, concern, and attending. All have been used to increase the frequency of desirable behavior by stutterers and are easily provided by clinicians in therapy sessions.

Events designed to reduce undesirable behavior have also taken numerous forms. Some of them, like loud noise and shock, are aversive and perhaps only useful in a laboratory situation. Others may be aversive but may carry information back to the stutterer that he has emitted a specific undesirable response. Saying words like "no," "that's wrong," and even "tree" (Cooper et al., 1970) have had a suppressive effect on undesirable responses. Other events, such as tabulating each instance of stuttering, having the stutterer reiterate his stuttered word (Carrier et al., 1969), and having the clinician repeat the word just stuttered (Blind et al., 1973) have also had the same suppressive effect. These types of events are more possible for the clinical situation and are easily provided by clinicians during therapy.

We cannot judge finally the effectiveness of any one of these contingent events in advance of their use in therapy. Such judgment requires a close and prompt scrutiny of whether changes in the desired direction are occurring. If such changes are not taking place, we look at each element of the paradigm; the evoking stimulus (if that is possible), the elements and properties of the responses we are trying to change, and the schedules, consistency, promptness, type, and forms of the contingent consequences we are providing. Such a systematic and operational approach to our clinical transactions should provide us with an understanding of our problems and enable us to arrange an appropriately individualized and effective therapeutic experience for each stutterer.

SUMMARY

Of primary importance in the development of an operant-based therapy program is the selection of a target response or target responses. These are the responses to be modified during therapy. Invaluable assistance in the selection process is given by the suggestions contained in many of the existing theories of stuttering. Subsequent to the selection of the target response, strategies for contingency management are planned. Here decisions are made about the clinician's response which is to be contingent upon the occurrence of a target response emitted by the stutterer. The success or failure of these strategies is assessed by recording changes in the frequency of occurrence of the target response with respect to a previous assessment made during a baseline period. In many respects, then, the development of a successful therapy program depends upon the search for a contingent response which, when utilized by the clinician, will result in desired changes in the frequency of the target response.

II

CLINICAL
APPLICATIONS
AND
CASE STUDIES

5

Introduction
to Part II

ORIENTATION

Part I dealt with the principles, the issues, and the controversies surrounding the clinical applications of operant procedures in the management of stuttering, and suggested many potential applications of operant principles to therapy. In the second part of the book we are concerned with actual studies and applications of the operant paradigm to the management of stuttering. Illustrative case studies will be cited from our work, as well as from the work of others.

Numerous studies of the application of operant procedures to stuttering have been reported. We can classify these studies into two categories: experimental and clinical. Most experimental studies are characterized by transience: stutterers are solicited and many times remunerated for participation in an experiment, and when the demands of the experimental design are satisfied, the stutterer's participation ends. No attempt is made to ameliorate stuttering and no such claim is made or implied. The stutterer serves merely as a data source. The value of the experiment lies in its yield of suggestions of the possible parameters that contribute to the acquisition, continuation, and reduction or elimination of stuttering. Suggestions given by experimenters about parameters and their value in controlling stuttering have often been used by clinicians in designing operant therapy programs. A case in point is the use of delayed auditory feedback (DAF) in the laboratory and the subsequent adoption of this technique in clinical programs. Though the experimenter can give potentially valuable suggestions to the clinician, the clinician must be wary of these suggestions. A well-designed experiment, with proper controls and adequate reliability and validity indices, which demonstrates a dramatic reduction in stuttering, may not establish the foundation of a good therapy program. We are aware of the susceptibility of stutterers to novelty and suggestion. Bloodstein's comment (Bloodstein, 1969), cited earlier, would testify to this point. Therefore, if any experimental results are to prove useful clinically, that confirmation must come from the clinician. Only in this way can verification be obtained. The clinician must possess a different kind of tenacity than is required of the experimenter. Of course, many times the dividing line between the laboratory and the clinical approach becomes blurred, as some experiments become longitudinal or long-term. Goldiamond (1965), for example, is viewed primarily as an experimenter, although his work resembles a clinician's because he saw his stutterers for extended periods of time. We would place our work on this middle ground and classify it as clinical research, meaning that we made a commitment to see the client for the time necessary to achieve desirable therapeutic results. While doing this, we simultaneously tested the efficacy of certain operant therapeutic strategies. Our clients were, of course, made aware of the experimental nature of the therapy they were about to receive.

While the experimental-clinical dichotomy is the major classification system for sorting operant applications, some subcategory systems are possible. A common one is to categorize studies according to the type of stimulation dispensed by the clinician contingent upon the occurrence of some response made by the stutterer. On this nominal dimension we find such category labels as noise, shock, delayed auditory feedback, time-out, point systems, token systems, response-cost, and verbal statements. Our own work is characterized by the last, in that we have primarily used verbal stimuli, contingent upon the evocation of certain predefined target responses made by the stutterer. The purpose of restricting ourselves to verbal stimuli is both theoretical and practical. On the theoretical level we hypothesized that restricting ourselves to verbal stimuli would permit us to work in an interpersonal setting, and, if fluency emerged in this setting, it might more readily generalize to other interpersonal settings outside of therapy than it would if the fluency emerged in the more contrived and socially remote laboratory setting. A practical reason for using verbal stimuli was that, if successful, the need for cumbersome, expensive, and complicated electronic circuitry would be eliminated. We have no *a priori* bias against electromechanical devices and physical stimuli but, if comparable results can be obtained without them, then we should proceed without them.

Evaluations and critiques about operant applications have involved a number of criteria: has stuttering been shown to be operant behavior? Does operant-based therapy lead to a reduction in stuttering? In short, is it successful? And how do operant therapies compare with the other therapeutic approaches extant? It is probably true that no one has yet demonstrated that stuttering is exclusively operant behavior. Much of the difficulty in demonstrating that stuttering is or is not operant is methodological, particularly in defining the discriminative stimuli that evoke stuttering. There is also a theoretical point that makes this issue somewhat of a classic issue, or an issue that is unanswerable but debatable for all time. Specifically, if in an experiment one finds that he is unsuccessful in manipulating stuttering by operant procedures he can hedge and state that he has not found the *right* contingent stimulus or discriminative stimulus. Whether or not stuttering is operant behavior is, therefore, of theoretical interest but not primary in application. Of major interest is the development of effective therapies for the management of stuttering. Reports published to date generally show that operant procedures have been successful in reducing stuttering under controlled conditions. However, in regard to the last criterion, we cannot say that operant-based therapies are superior to other therapies for stuttering. A number of reviews of operant therapy programs address themselves to the above criteria. Perkins (1971), Van Riper (1973), and Martin and Ingham (1973) present representative and recent evaluations. The evaluations are sobering, to say the least. For example, Martin and Ingham end their review by saying ". . . there is little reliable evidence to support the use of response contingent treatment procedures in stuttering therapy." Ingham, coupled this time with Andrews, in Ingham and Andrews (1973) makes a similar, less than enthusiastic evaluation, ". . . reports of behavior therapy for stuttering are disappointing in their absence of concern for appropriate and systematic evaluation of outcome." In general, we agree with these criticisms. The principal pleas of the reviewers are for tighter designs and measuring procedures so that favorable outcomes can indeed be attributed to the particular applied method. Moreover, they are concerned about the problem of carryover, where there is an even greater dearth of documentation of process and outcome.

In our own work the primary goal was to devise therapy programs using operant procedures for the purpose of assisting stutterers in becoming comfortably fluent. In the process we did not attempt to satisfy all the requirements of the ideal operant experiment. For example, we did not extend our baseline sessions over a period of weeks as a rigorous experimentalist might prefer and as is possible in the animal laboratory. There is, of course, a price for these departures, and it is that you cannot be as precise in attributing a particular effect to a particular paradigm. However, the consequences of these departures do not, we believe, obviate the use of operant procedures. We saw our task as one of establishing predictive validity and not construct validity. We were interested in designing therapy programs that would reliably enable stutterers to become fluent and not in designing programs that were isomorphically derived from the principles of operant conditioning.

The case studies reported in the following sections are representative of the clients, both adults and children, that were seen on the two research projects mentioned in the preface of this book.

PROCEDURES

In conducting these clinical studies certain general procedures were followed. Therapy sessions, all forty minutes in length, were conducted in small rooms furnished with a table and chairs. The rooms were equipped with microphones, video cameras, and hand-held electromechanical counters. The input to these devices was sent to recording devices in another room, eliminating the possibility of the client hearing relay noises. The hand-held electromechanical counters enabled the clinician to count response occurrences during therapy without any audible or visual detection by the client. In addition, in the recording room an assistant had available four additional electromechanical counters, and video and audio monitors. Thus, as a therapy session proceeded it was possible to simultaneously tally occurrences of six different responses. The results of these tabulations were recorded on digital counters and continuous recording polygraphs. Having the equipment arranged in this way was primarily for convenience as it permitted on-line analysis of the sessions. The results of each therapy session were punched on standard 80-column computer cards along with the clinician's comments. At any time these cards could be submitted and analyzed by a custom-written computer program that calculated percentages of occurrence of various therapy behaviors, and printed out both tabularly and graphically the session-by-session results of therapy. It is important to reiterate that the equipment and analytic procedures in our work were used primarily for convenience. Anyone with a tape recorder, a stopwatch, several hand-held tally counters, and paper and pencil could essentially duplicate our procedures.

Two measures routinely taken by us, irrespective of the therapy program and client, were the number of words uttered and the number of words stuttered. We divided the first measure into the second and multiplied by 100, yielding the percentage of words stuttered. Thus, if during a 40-minute session the stutterer uttered 4,000 words and stuttered 40 times, the percentage of stuttering would be 1 percent.

Periodic checks on the reliability of response judgment were made. It was possible to do some of these on line, particularly tests of interjudge reliability, since two people had available visual and auditory access to the therapy session and had independent means of counting the response in question. Intrareliability tests, of course, were done by replaying the recording of the therapy session. Reliability was calculated by taking a series of five-minute segments, obtaining at least two counts on each of these segments, and then correlating the distributions generated by the separate counts. Reliability correlation coefficients for stuttering never fell below .85. At times absolute measures of reliability were made by calculating the percentage of agreement between two judges. It is possible for two judges to generate high positive correlations but be consistently different in absolute numbers. When this occurred, absolute calculations were made in an attempt to determine the reasons for this systematic disparity.

Although the specific tactics described in these cases have been effective and appear promising, they are presented as vehicles for illustrating how the operant principles can be applied. The authors are aware of a number of other possible tactics that have not as yet been explored and are therefore not presented for discussion. We cannot emphasize strongly enough that it is the principles and not necessarily the tactics that we want the reader to take with him from this volume.

6

Evaluation
and Therapy
for Children

EVALUATION

IN SEARCH OF THE CAUSE

It is probably true that most of the information acquired in the evaluation of young stutterers is ignored in the planning and execution of therapy. This is due in part to the fact that no one as yet has been able to trace stuttering to an organic cause or physical pathology. Thus, questions about the medical history of parents and child will not yield critical information. For similar reasons, the developmental history of the child will, in most cases, yield information with only marginal value in the planning of therapy. Because stuttering is a disorder that emerges from the interpersonal dynamics of the child's environment, medical information is of secondary importance. It might be of interest to know that stuttering began after an accident or an illness, and indeed many times parents will fix the onset of stuttering to a single event at a specific time. Such fixation brings clarity to the situation and sufficiently answers the question often asked, alas, even by some clinicians, "When did *it* begin." Fixing the time and cause of onset also externalizes the cause. If, according to a parent, stuttering began when the child was injured after falling from a swing, the parent can attribute the stuttering to this external event and remove himself or herself from the matter. In like manner parents will attach the onset of stuttering to the time when their child was suffering from one of a number of childhood diseases. We said that these associations clarify the situation for the parents. We agree with the eighteenth-century philosopher David Hume that people have a psychological inclination for knowing or seeking the cause of a phenomenon. To wish that the cause be medical or due to physical trauma is another inclination that most of us possess. In general, people are less stigmatized by physical disorders than by behavioral ones. Finally, when we attribute a disorder to a physical cause we relieve ourselves of the responsibility for the disorder and the guilt that might accrue if the disorder were not externally caused. Thus, it seems we have all been victimized by events external to the dynamics of interpersonal relationships and the context of human interactions.

Clinicians at times tacitly agree with the parent's ideas about the cause of a child's stuttering. When asking questions about early medical history, clinicians encourage parents to recount illnesses and tragedies. The parents have come to see the clinician about their child's speech disorder and the speech clinician asks about medical problems. We feel it is not surprising that parents often then associate the speech disorder with a medical cause. When recalling medical traumas, parents will often reexperience some of the emotion surrounding these traumas. Clinicians will often show compassion and empathize with the parents. In doing so, it is possible that they give empathic acceptance to the parents' ideas. We do not object to the clinician demonstrating compassion. What we do object to is the clinician introducing topics in the evaluation session that may have little relevance to his management of the child, and that may bias his therapeutic approach.

Most clinicians would agree that stuttering has no physical or organic basis, but maintain nevertheless that physical traumas trigger psychological traumas and therefore are critical events in the acquisition of stuttering, albeit indirectly. We would agree that crises caused by illness and/or accident can change the psychological environment for periods of time, and that stuttering can emerge in this new environment. However, the child's interpersonal environment can be influenced by many factors besides those of physical pathology. For example, parents may report that their child began to stutter when a sibling was born, when they divorced, or when a grandparent died. Certainly such events are potential creators of stress and trauma, and both parents and clinicians alike are tempted to attach credibility to these attributions. Again clarity is gained, the cause is externalized, and possible guilt is lessened. We conclude, however, that spending time in an evaluation session looking for causes is not fruitful. It leads to speculations that may bias both clinician and family to believe stuttering is caused by some external event beyond anyone's control. Beliefs such as these tend to relieve participants of responsibility in therapy.

Based on our view that stuttering is acquired and maintained by the interpersonal dynamics between the child and his family, we hypothesize that evaluation time is best used in observing the child interact with his parents and people outside his family. Certain factors admittedly served as catalysts for the interaction patterns presented but it is the interaction itself that is of value. In observing a child and his parents together we can obtain information on the child's speech, particularly his fluency patterns; the parent's speech; and the parent-child interactions. In observing the child's speech we are concerned with the frequency, severity, and stability (consistency of occurrence) of stuttering. Of these three factors, we are particularly concerned with the stability of the child's stuttering patterns. We assume that a great degree of variance in the occurrence of the child's stuttering is of predictive value. By variance we mean that the child shows wide variance in the frequency and severity of stuttering depending on the listener and the situation. When the stuttered responses vary they are considered to be weaker. When the stuttered responses are consistent in their appearance irrespective of listener and situation, and when they are consistent in their frequency of occurrence and severity, then we assume that stuttering is more stable, stronger, and perhaps more resistant to remediation. The severity of the stuttering episode is also important and, like stability, is generally indicative of the strength of the stuttering: the more severe the stuttering blocks, the more resistant the response will be to remediation. Stability, more than episodic severity and general frequency of occurrence, is a measure of the strength of the response and a predictor of response to therapy. It is possible for a child to stutter severely but in a limited number of situations and with specific individuals. We would regard such a pattern as less stable than one where the child stuttered severely in all situations. Frequency of occurrence of stuttering is assessed in its relation to severity, stability, and occasions. Given a fixed severity and a constant stability, the greater the frequency of stuttering, the more resistant it is to modification.

As stability, severity, and frequency factors apply to the stuttering response, so do they apply to other behaviors that often occur in concert with the stuttering. Thus, hand movements, facial grimaces, and loss of eye contact will probably be predictive of a stronger, more stable stuttering pattern as the stability, severity, and frequency increase. It is these associated behaviors, sometimes called secondary symptoms, in combination with the frequency and severity of the stuttering response that are often used in categorizing childhood stuttering. There have been a number of proposed category systems: Bluemel's (1932) primary and secondary stages; Van Riper's (1954) primary, transitional, and secondary stages; Bloodstein's (1969) four phases in the development of stuttering; and Van Riper's (1971) more recent four tracks of stuttering development. These proposed stages of development are only loosely descriptive. As Bloodstein acknowledges (1969, p. 21), ". . . the outlines of the process of development are still far from clear."

THE INTERPERSONAL ENVIRONMENT

Observing the parents' speech seldom yields critical information related to the child's fluency problem. Occasionally, however, when seeing a parent and child interact, a parental speech pattern, having important implications for the assessment of the child's speech, is revealed. Parents can exhibit fluency and articulatory deviations that may be reflected in the speech of the child. When this is the case we have the possibility that the child's speech pattern is an imitation of the parents' speech. The child has learned his "mother tongue" and thus within his family constellation, he is normal.

The parent-child interaction reveals the most crucial information for us. Since we believe stuttering to be acquired in the child's interpersonal environment, and since the parents are the principals in the environment, it follows that contained in the parent-child interaction are the factors responsible for the acquisition and maintenance of stuttering. In operant conditioning terminology the contingencies controlling the child's stuttering exist in this interaction, be they reinforcing or punishing.

We applied our ideas about the importance of interaction when designing a speech evaluation for nine young stutterers.* This particular evaluation procedure was part of a larger experimental project that also involved "interaction" therapy. If, indeed, stuttering is acquired and maintained by certain parent-child interactions, then clues about what

---

* Much of the information presented in this section was reported in Egolf et al. (1972). Used by permission from the *J. of Speech and Hearing Disorders* and the authors.

maintains the stuttering, as well as clues about remediation, might be observed in the parent-child dyad. Consequently, our evaluation session consisted of two sections: first, the parent and child were placed in a room and asked to converse; and second, the clinician saw the child and sought to establish and maintain a dialogue with him. The first session was labeled the controlled waiting-room situation, or CWS; and the second, the therapy situation, or TS. During the evaluation, the two sessions were 30 and 25 minutes in length. All conversations were recorded and analyzed with respect to the frequency and severity of the child's stuttering in the CWS and TS and with respect to parent-child interaction in the CWS. We did not interview the parent and, therefore, did not obtain a case history. Some identifying information such as age, grade in school, and previous therapy was obtained from a short questionnaire the parents filled out before the evaluation session. All parents were informed about the experimental nature of our program, and all parent-child dyads knew that sessions were audio and/or video recorded.

Nine parent-child dyads were evaluated in this manner and all were accepted for therapy. Table 6.1 shows identifying information about the dyads as well as the frequency and severity of each child's stuttering in the CWS and TS. An inspection of Table 6.1 reveals that the nine children exhibited stuttering in varying degrees of frequency and severity. For the purpose of the child's sex identification, it was hoped that a parent of the same sex could accompany the child to therapy, but because of parents' work schedules, the parents who came to the evaluation sessions were also the parents free to accompany their children to therapy. Parent 9 specifically asked to come with his daughter, since he felt he needed to learn to talk to her.

Table 6.2 shows the results of our analysis of the parent-child interactions. The sessions were analyzed by viewing video tapes of the CWS and noting the qualitative aspects that most characterized the interaction in the session. An inspection of the table shows that Parent 1 was singularly accepting of her son, regardless of the content or manner of his speech. She did not seem to react differentially to him. Interaction patterns in Dyads 2 through 9 seemed more negative. Overall there was less spontaneous conversation on the part of either parent or child. Evident also were interruptions, interrogations, parents' refusals to talk about certain subjects, silent periods, and at times behavior characteristic of Piaget's collective monologue—that is, both parent and child talking but not taking each other into account. Parent 9 (father) was the only parent who reacted overtly to his child's stuttering. This he did by holding his hands over his ears, looking down, and shaking his head.

TABLE 6.1. Information from the Speech Evaluation Session.

Factor	Data (by subject)								
Subject	1	2	3	4	5	6	7	8	9
Age	13	6	8	13	9	11	7	5	13
Sex (parent)	F	F	F	F	F	F	M	F	M
Sex (child)	M	M	M	M	M	M	M	M	F
CWS stuttering frequency	14.3	5.7	2.6	13.0	5.3	3.7	12.0	3.8	2.1
TS stuttering frequency	23.8	25.7	2.5	12.8	6.8	4.5	5.1	4.3	1.9
CWS stuttering severity	2.51	1.34	2.11	2.21	2.15	2.15	2.09	1.23	1.25
TS stuttering severity	2.52	1.49	1.97	2.33	2.10	2.05	1.74	1.37	1.74
Previous therapy experience	2 yrs. school	None	2 yrs. school	2 mo. hosp. clinic	1 mo. school	3 yrs. school	6 mo. univ. clinic	None	None

Adapted from Egolf et al. (1972).

CWS = controlled waiting-room situation.

TS = therapy situation.

Stuttering frequency = number of words stuttered per 100 words uttered.

Stuttering severity = average rating based on a three-point scale ranging from 1 (mild) to 3 (severe).

CRITIQUE
OF THE SAMPLE EVALUATION PROCESS
FOR CHILDREN

The above represents the total evaluative process in this study. At least two things should be noticed. First, the path taken in designing this particular evaluation was one of many that could have been taken. However, rationales for the particular path are given, i.e., the particular choice is not a random one but is based on a belief that stuttering emerges from the child's patterns of interpersonal relations. Second, no case history was taken. Information is collected only on the parent-child behaviors presented at the time of the evaluation. It should also be noted that these evaluations focused on only a small aspect of the tactics suggested in Chapter Three. This was because our task was not one of differentiating normal dysfluency from stuttering. These were stutterers of long standing, who had been living with the label for several years.

It is quite possible that our assumptions about the interpersonal-relation genesis of stuttering are acceptable, but at the same time our derived evaluative procedures are less than adequate. It is apparent that we do not sample the child's interpersonal behavior to any degree of depth and breadth. Is 30 minutes of parent-child dialogue a sufficient sample from which inferences can be made? Should we not have observed the child speaking to both his parents, to siblings, and to other persons in the family constellations? Is the age of the child important to the validity of the interaction hypothesis? Perhaps. Once again we are reminded of the decision-making process and of the conflict between experimental and clinical considerations. Experimentally we would consider our evaluation inadequate; it would not pass the rigorous test of an adequate baseline. Clinically we considered it sufficient. Since we had planned to see the parent in subsequent therapy sessions, we were able to make a judgment on the representativeness of the parent-child interaction patterns. Moreover, since the child stuttered in the presence of the presenting parent, we assumed that particular parent to be involved somehow with the child's stuttering and specifically involved in the acquisition and maintenance of the child's stuttering. The validity of this evaluative procedure can be judged by the outcome of the therapy based on it. If our therapy (based on these evaluations) is effective, then the evaluative procedure is valid and worthwhile. If the outcome of therapy is poor, then these procedures should be reexamined.

THERAPY

In terms of operant logistics we can approach the young stutterer with a number of therapeutic strategies. We can seek directly to retard the extended conditioning or strengthening of stuttering; we can

TABLE 6.2. Description of Parent-Child Interactions.

Parent-Child Dyad	Description of Interaction	Examples	
1	Spontaneous speech by mother and child. Mother did not react differently to fluent or stuttering speech. Any topic acceptable for discussion.	Child:	I think I'll quit school when I'm old enough.
		Mother:	I thought you wanted to be a chemist.
2	Mother asked series of short questions. Child gave short, whiny answers. Child spoke spontaneously as fantasy character but did not interact with mother in fantasy role.	Mother:	Who sits in front of you in school?
		Child:	Nobody.
		Mother:	You're in the first row?
		Child:	Yeah. (Child grabs mike and goes into Dick Tracy routine.)
3	Mother showed verbal aggression. Child showed no spontaneous speech.	Mother:	Why don't you talk?
		Child:	(No response.)
		Mother:	Can't you talk?
		Child:	(No response.)
4	Lengthy silent periods. Mother verbally aggressive at times, asked many questions. Child gave short answers.	Mother:	Did Mr. Harvey say anything about plowing snow?
		Child:	No.
		Mother:	Do you think he'll let you?
		Child:	I don't know.
		Mother:	Do you think you can manage it?
		Child:	I don't know.
5	Mother constantly interrupted child, asked and answered her own questions.	Mother:	What are you going to do with that?
		Child:	Going to show ... (Here the child is interrupted).
		Mother:	You're going to give it to Mr. Johnson.
6	Mother and child verbally aggressive. Long periods of silence.	Mother:	You're supposed to be talking to me, not say "what stuff, huh?"
		Child:	I'm talking to you.
		Mother:	Well, tell me about what Houdini was.
		Child:	Well, he was a man—what do you think he was?
		Mother:	Just don't get smart—tell me what you read in the book.
7	Long periods of silence. Father asked series of questions. Child gave brief answers.	Father:	You must have a pile of homework, do you?
		Child:	No.
		Father:	Do you have any at all?
		Child:	(Nods.)
		Father:	What do you have?
		Child:	Um—English.
		Father:	Just English—what about math, spelling, and all those others?

TABLE 6.2. (Continued)

Parent-Child Dyad	Description of Interaction	Examples	
8	Mother degraded child, at times was verbally aggressive, enjoyed catching child in little logic traps. Long periods of silence. Many interruptions by parent.	Mother:	Do you remember this book?
		Child:	(Begins to talk but is interrupted.)
		Mother:	You don't remember Little Pearl?
		Child:	(Again interrupted.)
		Mother:	Answer me—do you remember Little Pearl?
		Child:	No.
		Mother:	Well, let's see—was Little Pearl a boy or a girl?
		Child:	Boy.
		Mother:	See, you do remember the book.
9	Father reacted to mild stuttering and aversive topics by holding hands over his ears, shaking his head, and sometimes saying, "No."	Child:	(Told father how girls rolled their skirts up to make them look like miniskirts.)
		Father:	No, no, no, don't tell me that. Does your mother know?

From Egolf et al. (1972). Used by permission from the *J. of Speech and Hearing Disorders* and the authors.

strengthen the already existent fluent patterns; we can seek indirectly to extinguish, suppress, or weaken stuttering patterns through environmental agents; we can teach a new form of fluent speech or a new, more acceptable form of stuttered speech; we can manipulate the environment in an attempt to eliminate the stimuli that evoke stuttering; or we can use the various approaches simultaneously and/or in sequence. Indeed, many times we use the *global approach* and like the unsure general or engineer we attack on all sides or overbuild because we are not certain about the strength of the enemy or the forces of nature. There is, of course, no a priori adverse reason for not taking the global approach. Simultaneous or combinatory attempts seem advisable as long as they are complementary in achieving the desired goal—a child who is comfortably fluent. Traditionally we see this complementarity in therapy for children when parent-counseling sessions are conducted concurrent with individual interview sessions with the child.

Because the child-stutterer has stuttered for a shorter time than the "case-hardened" adult, we assume that the strength of his stuttering-response repertoire is weaker. In addition, we assume the strength of stuttering varies widely among child stutterers. This further assumption is based on the observations that we make about the frequency and severity of stuttering behaviors and associated behaviors, and the length of time the child has been exhibiting the behaviors. These gradations of strengths and weaknesses direct our approaches to therapy with children, particularly our initial approaches.

Wendell Johnson has written that stuttering begins in the parent's ear, not in the child's mouth, and that what is often labeled stuttering is essentially normal behavior, because in the course of learning speech and language the majority of children exhibit it (see Bloodstein, 1969, p. 43). If we accept Johnson's conclusions, we will be most sensitive to an approach that seeks to eliminate the acquisition of stuttering or to arrest any further development of stuttering. Such an approach is manifest in therapy that consists solely of parent-counseling. Here parents are advised that the behavior of their child is essentially normal or developmental in nature, and that this behavior will dissipate if they do not react to it in a way that will signal to the child that he is doing something wrong. Such signals merely trigger a cyclical series of apprehensions and speech dysfluencies, and if continued the child may develop into a stutterer. Parenthetically it may be noted that some earlier and incorrect transmissions of Johnson's ideas from clinicians to parents were often in the form of a curt directive, "Just ignore it." Parents remained quiet about their child's stuttering, but their actions spoke louder than words, and stuttering developed. We believe that now most clinicians are aware of the persuasiveness of both verbal and nonverbal means of communication.

The strength of the stuttering response in the normally dysfluent child as characterized by Johnson would logically be zero, since by definition the child is not stuttering. Some may even feel obliged by this logic to exclude such children from the category of stuttering. We feel no such compulsion because we believe that when a child approaches or falls into the category of normal dysfluency, efforts should be made to prevent the acquisition of stuttering or to arrest and reverse its development. The recipients of these efforts are the parents. This would be true even if stuttering were not acquired as Johnson suggests. While we consider Johnson's thesis to be valid we do not think it accounts for the way in which stuttering develops in all children. We hold that there may be many mechanisms for the acquisition of stuttering in children. One such mechanism may be profound verbal or physical punishment. The child may be punished verbally or nonverbally by the parent when he is going to speak, actually speaking, or immediately after speaking. It may be important to differentiate parental reactions that are mildly aversive and provide information to the child about his speech from reactions that are profoundly aversive and may reduce the child's perceptions of self-worth and parental love. The first type of event may serve to reduce stuttering or dysfluency and is compatible with the "punishment" studies from the operant laboratories. The second type of event may result in extreme emotional reactions that interfere with ongoing operant speaking behavior. Regardless of the mechanism responsible for acquisition the initial approaches are almost identical. Concern is with the processes of prevention, arrest, and reversal; and the parent is the recipient of treatment.

With the child in the advanced stages of stuttering, a variety of the above operant logistics is often employed. To be recognized of course is the fact that the development of stuttering is not a discrete, abrupt transition but one of continuity. The child who demonstrates overt stuttering behaviors such as grimaces, tonic and clonic body movements, and loss of eye contact, may still have dysfluency as well as fluency free of these overt behaviors. Such variability in behavior suggests that the child may possess many of these behaviors in low strength. This variability is manifest many times as listeners vary. The child may be fluent with a grandparent but not with a parent and vice versa.

When a child's stuttering seems to be low in strength, that is, the stuttering is highly variable in occurrence, it seems advisable to use some of the strategies associated with prevention, arrest, and reversal. Here focus is on the parent in the form of counseling, and environmental manipulation, in an attempt to reduce the stresses placed on the child. Basic rationales for these strategies rest on the notion that direct therapeutic action with a child can convince him of the idea that something is indeed wrong with him, and subsequently he will act in harmony with this belief. Convincing evidence for the child can be nonverbal; for instance, he is taken somewhere other children are not, like a speech clinic, a speech class, or a hospital setting. Or, it can be verbal; for instance, a clinician tells him why he has been brought to this particular clinic. As courtrooms and hospitals can evoke feelings of guilt and illness, so may speech clinics evoke "something is wrong with me" attitudes in children. By these comments we do not want to imply that direct intervention with the child should be avoided. Children, particularly those who have advanced beyond the transitory stage, are aware that something is wrong, and for parents and other adults to ignore this places a double burden on the child. The child knows that something is wrong but he must not let anyone know that he knows. A qualitative rule of thumb for clinicians would seem to be to obtain the maximum gains therapeutically with a minimum amount of direct intervention.

With the child whose stuttering appears invariably and predictably and therefore is in great strength, a variety of approaches can be taken, including, most usually, direct intervention. Direct intervention means that the child is scheduled and seen regularly in the therapeutic process. Parents may or may not be regular participants in therapy. Any one or any combination of the logistics mentioned at the outset of this section can be used with these children. Our own approach to therapy with the child stutterer is as follows: After concluding an evaluation session that includes both parent and child, a decision is made about the strength of the child's stuttering. If the child does not stutter, as evidenced by his behavior, or his age (or his parents have unrealistic expectations of how he should speak), parent counseling is the primary approach, with intermittent or no further observations of the child. For the remaining children, those children who do stutter, we have attempted to modify stuttering with a single, accommodating therapeutic program. The program is tied into the evaluation process described earlier in this chapter. We assumed that stuttering emerges in the child's interpersonal environment and that this environment includes primarily the child and his parents. The parent of the stuttering child is in a state of equilibrium and this equilibrium serves to maintain stuttering. The goal of therapy is to disturb this equilibrium so that a new equilibrium can be established, one which does not include stuttering. By a two-step process we attempt to create this new equilibrium, first in a situation involving the clinician and the child. Then, we introduce the parent into the situation (see Table 6.3).

TABLE 6.3.   Schematic Outline of the Therapy Program.

A 15-minute CWS (controlled waiting-room situation) session is conducted before therapy in both stages.

Stage	Participants	Clinician's Role	Criterion for Moving On
1	Clinician and child	a. Interact with child in a manner different from that of parent. b. Demonstrate to child his improved speech by replaying fluent audio samples.	Less than 1 percent stuttering in one session.
2	Clinician, child, and parent	a. Maintain interpersonal role assumed in Stage 1. b. Provide a vicarious speaking model for parent. c. Share speaking time equally with parent.	Fluency with clinician and parent.

From Egolf et al. (1972). Used by permission from the *J. of Speech and Hearing Disorders* and the authors.

The clinician disturbs the assumed equilibrium by reacting to the child in a manner opposite to that of the parent. For example, if the parent constantly interrupts the child, the clinician avoids interruptions; if the parent refuses to talk about certain topics, the clinician listens to the child talk about these topics. The therapeutic strategy becomes a mirror image of the interaction observed during the evaluation.

Following are details for incorporating our basic assumption into a therapeutic program.* Application of this program to the nine parent-child dyads is also included. These are the same children whose evaluations were discussed in the previous section.

A 15-minute controlled waiting-room situation (CWS) preceded each therapy session. Observation of the parent and child before each session yielded information on the stability of the interaction patterns observed in the evaluation session and provided an index of the extent to which fluency gains acquired in therapy were generalizing outside of therapy.

Therapy was conducted in two stages. In Stage 1 our goal was to evoke fluent conversation from the child. We decided that this would be achieved when the child, during one 40-minute therapy session, stuttered on one word or no words for each 100 words uttered. The attempt to evoke fluency was based on applying our primary strategy outlined above, that is, with the clinician assuming an interpersonal role different from that of the parent. Strategies derived for each child are contained in Table 6.4. This table viewed in conjunction with Table 6.3 shows the interpersonal role of the clinician in contrast with that of the parent. As there were commonalities in parent-child interactions, so there were commonalities in therapeutic strategies. With Children 3 through 9, the clinician attempted to create an atmosphere conducive to spontaneous conversation by displaying attention to what the child had to say. No topic was forbidden. With Child 1, whose mother seemed to be most accepting of the content and manner of her son's speech, the clinician was less accepting, particularly of the child's stuttering. The clinician had this child "experiment" with various ways of talking, which resulted in more fluent and comfortable speech. The child was then asked to listen to audiotape playbacks of his "experiments," especially the ones producing fluency. He then evaluated these samples to identify the "things he did" that resulted in fluency. Child 2 was fluent in the evaluation session when he portrayed a fictional character. In therapy we tried to phase the "fictional" fluency into the real world by using puppets and gradually changing the roles given to the puppets from fictional to real-life char-

---

* From Egolf et al. (1972). Used by permission from the *J. of Speech and Hearing Disorders* and the authors.

TABLE 6.4. Clinician's Manner of Interaction with the Children.
"Reward" means the clinician's expressed interest in what the child said;
he usually asked a question that required the child to give more information
on a topic the child initiated.

Child	Manner	Example
1	Do not accept stuttering. Have child discover new way of talking.	Clinician had child experiment with various ways of talking to find a way that was easy for the child to produce fluency.
2	Use puppets to teach child social interaction and to have him experience fluent speech in dialogue.	Clinician began by having dialogue while he and the child had puppets. Initially both clinician and child were fantasy characters. Gradually fantasy characters were changed to real characters and puppets were removed.
3	Reward spontaneous verbal output.	Talked about scouting. Discussed badges, projects, stars, camping trips, and bivouacs.
4	Reward verbal output. Give opportunity for success (in verbal and nonverbal tasks) and praise it.	Talked about football. Went over highlights of previous Sunday's game. Set up various offenses and defenses on the blackboard.
5	Do not interrupt child. Reward verbal output.	Went into great detail about music, since child played trumpet and drums. Child "taught" clinician about beats, measures, whole notes, scales, and keys.
6	Reward nonaggressive verbal output.	Child brought in his collection of Hot Wheel cars. Discussed various track layouts. Child wrote a play that was presented in his school assembly. Casting, rehearsals, and production were discussed.
7	Give acceptance for ideas and thoughts, and reward verbal output.	Child brought his guitar to therapy. He explained strings, chords, frets, keys, and tuning. Child played and sang a few songs, which evoked a lengthy discussion about the differences between speaking and singing.
8	Give praise for coming to therapy and reward verbal output.	Clinician greeted child each week with "I'm glad to see you" or "I was looking forward to today." Talked about school and camping.
9	Listen to child. Be accepting of whatever topic she introduces. Discuss word and situation fears.	Talked about latest trends in the length of skirts and in pop music. Talked about certain words and situations the girl feared. Child talked about her parents' attitudes and contrasted them with her own.

From Egolf et al. (1972). Used by permission from the *J. of Speech and Hearing Disorders* and the authors.

acters. When fluent speech was evoked, audio playbacks of the fluent samples were presented to the child to demonstrate to him that he was able to do a "good job at talking."

Our goal in Stage 2 of therapy was to generalize the fluency obtained in the therapy situation (TS) to the environment, or, more specifically, to the parent, and to have this fluency maintained. We attempted to achieve this by introducing the parent into the TS and alternately having the clinician and parent talk with the child. The clinician maintained his basic interpersonal role as outlined in Table 6.3. We hoped that arranging the TS in this way would activate two processes: generalization, in the traditional learning theory sense, and vicarious learning by the parent. We predicted that a response, such as fluency from a child, evoked in the presence of a stimulus, such as a clinician, would generalize most readily to another listener, such as the parent, if the clinician were present. Our major assumptions suggest that when the child acquires increased fluency the parent must make corresponding changes in his behavior if the dyad is to achieve a new equilibrium. To this end the clinician can serve as a model and teach the parent new ways of reacting to his child.

RESULTS OF THERAPY

Table 6.5 shows the results of the initial application of our method for 13 months. Data for both stages of therapy, as well as intrastage data, are given. Six of the nine subjects reached Stage 2 of therapy, meaning that they were fluent at least 99 percent of the time in the TS. All subjects, except Child 8 in the CWS, experienced some increased fluency.

Although the children consistently stuttered more with their parents than with the clinician in Stage 1, over time their fluency with their parents increased. Apparently, some generalization was occurring. The Stage 2 data provide more impressive evidence for generalization. In Stage 2 when the parent is in the TS and the child divides his speaking time between the clinician and the parent, stuttering frequency remains low. In short, the influence of the clinician is pervasive. The fluency evoked in his presence generalized to the parent.

Table 6.6 lists data from the final session. A comparison of this table with Table 6.1 shows that almost all the children experienced decreases in stuttering frequency and severity. Where this was not the case or where changes were only marginal, we noted an associated poor attendance record.

Children 1, 3, 5, 6, 7, and 9 were discharged because they completed the program. Of the remaining three children, one moved from the area

TABLE 6.5.   Mean Frequencies of Stuttering.

| Child | | Stage 1 | | | | Stage 2 | | | |
| | | First Half | | Second Half | | First Half | | Second Half | |
		CWS	TS	CWS	TS	CWS	TS	CWS	TS
1	M	15.1	9.4	12.1	1.5	7.9	0.5	–	–
	SD	2.9	6.6	5.3	1.4	5.7	0.9	–	–
	N	12	12	14	14	4	4	–	–
2	M	5.0	3.5	4.5	2.5	–	–	–	–
	SD	1.1	2.1	1.8	0.8	–	–	–	–
	N	10	10	11	11	–	–	–	–
3	M	2.6	1.1	4.5	1.5	2.4	0.5	2.7	0.6
	SD	1.1	0.7	3.0	1.1	2.3	0.8	2.7	0.8
	N	11	11	11	11	15	15	15	15
4	M	16.7	9.8	14.7	8.0	–	–	–	–
	SD	2.6	5.5	6.1	3.1	–	–	–	–
	N	11	11	11	11	–	–	–	–
5	M	4.4	2.9	3.8	2.1	2.0	1.2	–	–
	SD	1.3	2.3	9.0	0.8	2.2	1.9	–	–
	N	8	8	8	8	6	6	–	–
6	M	4.3	2.9	3.3	3.0	1.9	0.6	0.5	0.4
	SD	1.1	1.0	3.7	2.6	1.3	0.2	0.7	0.6
	N	12	12	12	12	7	7	10	10
7	M	9.4	3.2	7.1	2.2	5.4	1.3	3.8	1.3
	SD	4.8	1.8	2.0	1.6	4.6	1.7	3.5	1.6
	N	11	11	11	11	15	15	12	12
8	M	4.4	2.7	5.1	2.0	–	–	–	–
	SD	1.2	1.0	1.5	0.5	–	–	–	–
	N	6	6	7	7	–	–	–	–
9	M	2.8	1.6	2.7	1.2	1.5	0.6	1.0	0.3
	SD	1.0	0.5	0.6	0.5	1.4	0.9	1.0	0.4
	N	7	7	7	7	15	15	11	11

From Egolf et al. (1972). Used by permission from the *J. of Speech and Hearing Disorders* and the authors.

CWS = controlled waiting-room situation.

TS = therapy situation.

M = mean number of words stuttered per each 100 words uttered.

SD = standard deviation.

N = numbers of sessions.

and two were given the opportunity to stay in the program. The parents of the latter chose instead to have their children treated in their respective schools. We were able to reevaluate five of the six children who completed the program. Table 6.7 contains information from these reevaluations. A comparison of Table 6.6 with Table 6.7 shows that, in general, therapeutic results were maintained and somewhat improved in both the CWS and TS.

To determine whether or not the clinician served as a positive

TABLE 6.6. Data from Final Therapy Session for
Each Child.

Child	Stuttering Frequency		Stuttering Severity	
	CWS	TS	CWS	TS
1	1.1	1.0	2.32	1.88
2	3.6	1.3	1.41	1.51
3	3.1	2.0	2.01	1.00
4	8.4	5.9	2.26	2.32
5	4.1	3.7	1.89	1.65
6	2.7	0.0	2.00	1.75
7	9.7	1.5	1.23	1.00
8	4.7	2.8	1.28	1.24
9	0.0	0.0	0.00	0.00

From Egolf et al. (1972). Used by permission from the
J. of Speech and Hearing Disorders and the authors.

CWS = controlled waiting-room situation.

TS = therapy situation.

speaking model in Stage 2 of therapy, a review session was held for those parents whose children reached Stage 2 and were later discharged from therapy. The ostensible reason for this review was to demonstrate to the parent, by having him view videotapes recorded in the early and final stages of therapy, the progress his child had made. A more important reason was to determine whether or not the parent had learned to interact more favorably with his child. The parents' comments during the

TABLE 6.7. Frequency of Stuttering for Five
Children Reevaluated after Discharge.

Child	Stuttering Frequency		Elapsed Time Since Discharge (in months)
	CWS	TS	
3	0.0	1.5	2
5	4.2	3.7	9
6	0.6	1.8	5
7	0.3	0.8	5
9	0.0	0.0	8

From Egolf et al. (1972). Used by permission from the
J. of Speech and Hearing Disorders and the authors.

CWS = controlled waiting-room situation.

TS = therapy situation.

All entries refer to number of words stuttered for each 100
uttered.

viewing were recorded. Some sample statements are possible evidence of vicarious learning:

Parent 3:   I think the encouragement and praise you gave John was marvelous. It meant a lot to him.

Parent 5:   I was surprised that you let Phillip talk about whatever he wanted to talk about.

Parent 7:   You encouraged him to go into detail about any given subject. Steven does well when he's encouraged.

Parent 9:   In the first tape, I find myself not treating her [Child 9] with the proper amount of consideration; maybe not as much as I would an outsider.

FURTHER APPLICATION

After the initial testing of our program with the nine parent-child dyads, we applied the program in an elementary school system. Children in seven elementary schools were screened and 13 stutterers were identified. Both evaluation and therapy procedures were intended to be identical to those in the previous application. Children were observed speaking with their parents and hypothesized maintaining factors of

TABLE 6.8.   **Results of Speech Evaluation Session for Thirteen Elementary School Children.**

Child	Age	Child's Sex	Parent's Sex	Percentage of Words Stuttered	
				CWS	TS
1	10	M	F	2.70	1.66
2	10	M	F	1.95	2.01
3	10	M	F	7.11	8.03
4	9	M	F	3.30	2.07
5	7	M	F	4.72	2.78
6	13	F	F	3.43	4.66
7	11	M	F	3.92	1.87
8	13	M	F	7.69	8.57
9	9	M	F	4.56	5.03
10	6	M	F	16.06	12.33
11	7	M	F	17.31	9.30
12	9	M	*	2.63	5.39
13	9	F	F	1.97	2.10

From Shames and Egolf (1971).

CWS = controlled waiting-room situation.

TS = therapy situation.

*Child was an orphan. Teacher conversed with child in CWS.

stuttering were extracted from these interactions. From these factors, moreover, therapeutic strategies were derived. Table 6.8 gives the results of the speech evaluation for these children and Table 6.9 summarizes the parent-child interactions and the derived therapeutic strategies.

Inspection of Table 6.8 shows stuttering frequencies ranging from

TABLE 6.9. Hypothesized Factors Maintaining Stuttering and Derived Therapeutic Strategies for Thirteen Parent-Child Dyads Seen in Elementary Schools.

Parent-Child Dyad	Hypothesized Maintaining Factors	Derived Therapeutic Strategies
1	Mother demanding and authoritative. Asking questions with little time for answers.	Reinforce initiation of topic. Give opportunity for lengthy utterances.
2	Mother makes curt statement. Does not react to child's answers.	Show interest in what the child says. Put remarks in statement form.
3	Parent aggressive and demanding. Stress on superior achievement.	Accept all levels of performance. Evaluate speech performance.
4	Parent reacted to nonfluencies rather than content of child's speech. Child aware of nonfluencies.	Praise all utterances. No reaction to nonfluencies.
5	Rapid speech by mother and child. Few silent periods.	Speak slowly. Silent period before response.
6	Parent accepts stuttering.	Do not accept stuttering. Reinforce fluent speech.
7	Child aware of stuttering. Parent does not react to stuttering.	Reinforce insight statements about stuttering. Demand fluent speech.
8	Mother passive. Child dominating conversation.	Place child on program of mild verbal punishment for stuttering responses.
9	Mother aggressive. Interaction primarily question and answer.	Reinforce topics initiated by child. Encourage child to talk and show interest in topic.
10	Parent intolerant of child and of therapy situation.	Reinforce child for coming to therapy and for all utterances.
11	Parent aggressive. Dominated conversation giving child little time for response.	Reinforce utterances and fluent speech.
12	No parent available in this case. Child was in residence.	Place child on program of mild punishment for stuttering responses and reinforce fluent speech.
13	Parent directed conversation and censored topics discussed.	Encourage child to speak freely. Reinforce fluent speech.

From Shames and Egolf (1971).

1.66 percent for Child 1 in the TS to 17.31 percent for Child 11 in the CWS. Parental interaction patterns as seen in Table 6.9 are generally negative, as they were with the nine parents reported on previously. Because Child 12 was an orphan, he talked with a teacher in the CWS and this interaction was not analyzed.

The screening, identification, and therapy for stutterers in the school system were carried out during one school term. The children were seen for therapy on a weekly basis. It was found that parents were not able to attend each therapy session as they did in our initial application. This was due mainly to their unavailability during the school hours, whereas parents in the initial application were seen at their convenience, mostly during the evening. We proceeded with the program nevertheless and the results of the application are contained in Table 6.10. For comparison, both beginning percentages of stuttering and final session information are given.

All children showed decreases in both the TS and CWS sessions. It is important to note that the decreases in stuttering frequency were gradual. Therefore, the final session data seen in Table 6.10 is representative of the final sessions, and the initial session data is representative of the early sessions. Thus there is evidence that the decreases in stuttering

TABLE 6.10.   Initial and Final Session Percentages of Stuttering for Thirteen Elementary School Children.

Child	Initial Session		Final Session		Number of Sessions
	CWS	TS	CWS	TS	
1	2.70	1.66	0.12	0.00	21
2	1.95	2.01	0.00	0.54	12
3	7.11	8.03	0.64	0.22	20
4	3.30	2.07	0.00	0.24	21
5	4.72	2.78	0.35	0.36	15
6	3.43	4.66	1.09	1.20	13
7	3.92	1.87	1.21	1.14	14
8	7.69	8.57	0.00	0.45	16
9	4.56	5.03	1.36	1.16	13
10	16.06	12.33	5.48	3.45	13
11	17.31	9.30	4.55	1.64	13
12	2.63	5.39	1.18	1.11	12
13	1.97	2.10	0.29	0.53	10

From Shames and Egolf (1971).
CWS = controlled waiting-room situation.
TS = therapy situation.

were stable and not episodic. We concluded on the basis of the two applications of the program that our thesis, that the acquisition and maintenance of stuttering is a function of the child's interpersonal relations, has merit. Some differences in the two applications, however, forced us to think about the nature of the interpersonal dynamics as controllers of stuttering and fluency. In the first application, parents attended all sessions and were part of the therapy in Stage 2 of the program. We assumed that they learned how to react more positively to their children. Parent reports testified in support of this assumption.

In the second application parents participated far less and none actually participated in the TS in Stage 2, where both parent and clinician talk with the child. It therefore can be concluded that little opportunity was available for vicarious learning as it was in the first application. Nonetheless, final session data as reported in Table 6.10 reveal that the children experienced increased fluency levels both with the clinician and the parent. Fluency acquired by the children in therapy did seem to generalize to CWS or the parent-child setting. These findings raised many questions. For example, does a child of a parent who exhibits an overall negative interpersonal reaction pattern change his parent's pattern when he becomes fluent? If not, does the parent's interactional behavior lose its assumed controlling properties, permitting the fluency pattern to be maintained? To begin to answer these questions we felt it most imperative to be able to characterize more rigorously the parent-child interactions. To this point our characterizations were impressionistic and global.

PARENT-CHILD INTERACTION ANALYSIS

In an effort to make our analysis of the parent-child interaction more precise and objective we constructed an interaction analysis scale (Shames and Egolf, 1971). The method was based in part on the ideas of Haim Ginott as represented in his book, *Between Parent and Child* (Ginott, 1969), and in part on our own clinical experience. Our method yields a quantitative profile of the parent's verbal behavior when talking to his child and shows the distribution of the parent's verbal statements across 35 thematic categories, 17 positive and 18 negative. A positive statement is one that encourages mutual respect between parent and child, and indicates acceptance of the child's feelings and ideas. A negative statement is one that fosters distrust, hostility, aggression, or silence. These positive and negative categories are presented in Tables 6.11 and 6.12. In using the interaction system, we placed each parental statement uttered in dialogue with the child in one of the content categories.

TABLE 6.11. Positive Thematic Language Categories.

Language Category	Definition	Example
1. Positive Question	Question that encourages vocalization	"What did you do in school today?"
2. Positive Advice	Advice preceded by understanding	"If you are well rested you are stronger. That's why you should go to bed early."
3. Positive Praise	Praise aimed at the child's actions or deeds instead of his personality	"You did a fine job washing the car."
4. Positive Comparison	Comparison that indicates understanding	"Sometimes even I am afraid of the dark."
5. Event-Feeling	Statement that takes into account the child's feeling when he relates an event	If the child says that the teacher yelled at him in school, a good event-feeling statement is, "I guess you were quite embarrassed."
6. Sequitur	Statement that follows in content the direction of the child's conversation	
7. Positive Criticism	Criticism preceded by understanding	"I know you are restless but you can't pull the curtain in the clinic."
8. Verbal Lubricant	Statement that demonstrates the listener's attentiveness and interest	"That's interesting—tell me more."
9. Mirrors Personality	Statement that reflects the child's apparent feelings	"I see you are angry now."
10. Permits Ambivalence	Statement that shows acceptance of bipolar feelings	"Sometimes you just don't like your brother."
11. Identifies Reasons for Emotions	Statement that helps the child focus his emotions	"It looks like you might be kicking things around because your brother got a letter today and you didn't."
12. Understands Feelings	Statement that helps the child accept a feeling	"I know you would like to receive a letter, too."
13. Humor	Laughter without a trace of sarcasm	
14. Qualifying	Statements preceded by "If," "I think," "I guess"	
15. Information	Statement that presents new information	"While you were at school, Grandma called."
16. Parent's Thoughts and Feelings	Statement that shows the parent identifying his thoughts and feelings and the reasons for them	
17. Other	Residual category for a positive statement that does not fit easily into the other positive categories	

Adapted from Shames and Egolf (1971).

TABLE 6.12. Negative Thematic Language Categories.

Language Categories	Definition	Example
1. Negative Question	Question that causes the child to lie, that can be answered by a "yes" or "no," or that has an obvious answer	"Do you like your teacher?"
2. Negative Advice	Advice not preceded by understanding	
3. Negative Praise	Praise that is global and not directed to a specific act	"You're just such a good boy."
4. Negative Comparison	Comparison that attacks the personality	"Your brother never had a D in math."
5. Event-Feeling	Statement that shows reaction to the event rather than the feeling	If the child says he was yelled at in school, a negative response is, "You must have been bad."
6. Non-Sequitur	Self-explanatory	
7. Negative Criticism	Criticism not preceded by understanding	
8. Insult	Self-explanatory	
9. Sarcasm	Self-explanatory	
10. Prophesying	Statement that makes a dire prediction	"If you keep rubbing your eyes, you will go blind."
11. Threat	Self-explanatory	"If you don't shut up, you're going to get it when we get home."
12. Bribe	Self-explanatory	"If you are good, we'll stop at the store."
13. Dictates Feelings	Statement that tells the child how to feel	"You should be happy."
14. Dictates Action	Statement that directs the child's behavior	"Look at the man when you talk."
15. Denial	Statement in which the parent denies something without explanation	"Your father wasn't mad at you."
16. Aborts	Statement that seemingly shows acceptance but by its manner disrupts conversation	"That's very interesting but now I want to tell you something."
17. Interruption	Self-explanatory	
18. Other	A residual category for a negative statement that does not fit easily into the other negative categories	

Adapted from Shames and Egolf (1971).

In the first application of this interaction analysis system we and Kasprisin-Burrelli (1972) hypothesized that if parental interactions were indeed instrumental in maintaining stuttering, then parents of stuttering children should display interaction patterns different from those of parents of nonstutterers, and that parents of stuttering children should interact differently if their children acquired fluent speech. Both hypotheses were confirmed. It was found that (1) a significantly greater number of positive statements were uttered by control parents than by parents of stutterers, and (2) that a significantly greater number of positive statements were uttered by parents of stutterers at the end of their children's therapy than at the beginning.

FUTURE ANALYSES

We are aware, of course, that our research does not categorically tie the emergence and amelioration of stuttering to the parent-child interaction environment. To reach such a conclusion we would have to show precisely how certain parental responses were of such consequence, and that they predictably resulted in the emergence of stuttered speech or fluency in the children. To be confirmed, such a conclusion would have to be supported by a number of verified predictions. Included here would be: that parents of a stuttering child interact differently with their nonstuttering children; that positive parental interaction results in fluency; if it is a cause-and-effect relationship, that the child's fluency does not change parental interaction but that parental interaction affects the child's fluency; that in reported cases of spontaneous remission of stuttering we would find the cooccurrence of a positive interpersonal relation. These are only a few of the hypotheses that can potentially be generated.

At the same time, however, the existence of untested hypotheses and questions need not separate the clinician from the information garnered on parent-child interactions and stuttering. We can say without hesitation that when parents react to their children in more positive ways the tendency is for fluency to emerge. Appropriate large-scale research may reveal that such positive verbal interactions early in life may function as a preventative for stuttering. Application need not await the answer to every experimental question.

SUMMARY

In this chapter we proposed that the evaluation of a child suspected of stuttering should be based on certain theoretical assumptions about the acquisition and maintenance of stuttering. The evaluation, furthermore, should yield findings that are instrumental in the subsequent management of the child if a problem exists. An evaluation and a management program meeting these criteria were presented. The basic assumption was that stuttering emerges in the child as a result of his attempts to achieve balance or equilibrium in his interpersonal relations. The stuttering is maintained for similar reasons. Strategies for therapy were also derived from this assumption. Most notable among these was having the clinician assume an interpersonal role opposite that observed in the parent. The rationale was that if stuttering indeed were maintained because of some balance that emerged in the child's interpersonal relationships, perhaps stuttering might change if the interpersonal dynamics were changed. Support for the basic assumption and the derivative strategies was found. Further research in this area of evaluation and therapy may enable clinicians to become more effective in both the amelioration and prevention of stuttering.

7

··

Evaluation
and Therapy
for Adults

EVALUATION

While speech evaluation is often required to determine whether or not the child is actually a stutterer, seldom is this decision difficult to make with the adult stutterer. His problem has been diagnosed and repeatedly confirmed through the years. The typical adult stutterer has a long history of both stuttering and therapy. Many times he challenges the clinician by recounting his therapeutic history. He recites a requiem for the techniques that have failed. He is obviously skeptical about the clinician's ability to help him.

As discussed in Chapter Three, evaluations for the adult stutterer have traditionally included detailed history taking, testing, and analysis. There has been little use of such information in determining whether or not the adult is a stutterer, or in planning therapy. The critical question is, of course, how is the information garnered in an evaluation session to be used in making the diagnosis or in planning therapy.

Some of the information presented in this chapter appeared in Shames et al. (1969) . Used by permission from the *J. of Speech and Hearing Disorders* and the authors.

A clinician who utilizes operant techniques is more interested in observing behavior than he is in hearing reports about behavior. The latter is second-order information filtered through the sensory-perceptual-cognitive system of its supplier, while the former is first order and more objective. And, too, it is the latter that is most often the target for therapeutic manipulation. Therefore, the primary goal for us in an evaluation session is to observe performance and not a meta-performance or a report about performance.

Even with this narrowed focus there remains still a large variety of observational approaches we can take with adult stutterers. Chapter Three lists some of the potential approaches. The approach we used in evaluating adult stutterers involved but one principal instruction, "I would like you to talk for 40 minutes." We focused on two categories of behavior: frequency of stuttering and thematic content. No case histories were taken, no questions were asked about any particular content introduced by the client, and no questions asked by the client were answered by the clinician during this 40-minute period. Thus the stutterer was totally responsible for composing some narrative; he was unable to passively answer the clinician's questions. The 40-minute monologue provided us the opportunity to observe how the stutterer talked and what he chose to talk about. This evaluation tactic was directly related to our general aims in therapy. We evaluated only those behaviors we were prepared to manage in therapy.

FORM AND CONTENT

Form refers to how the stutterer talks, *content* refers to what he talks about. In monitoring a large number of evaluation sessions with adult stutterers, we found that the most discriminating categories of information for characterizing stutterers were the form-content categories. Those stutterers who fell in the form category were those whose speech was dominated by the traditional overt characteristics of stuttering such as repetitions, struggle, and prolongations. The content stutterers were those whose speech was relatively free of the overt manifestations of stuttering but who talked about fears of stuttering, fears of being found out, feelings of victimization, and so on. The form stutterer's speech is so populated with interruptions that intelligibility is hampered. The content stutterer produces utterances relatively free of such interruptions. In fact we have seen some stutterers who produced 40 minutes of fluent speech. However, in most instances, stutterers reveal varying combinations of both characteristics.

We have found this form-content dichotomy a useful one in constructing therapy programs for adults. The form stutterer, who produces only wreckages of phrases, needs to be given the experience of fluency. In this way the stutterer can receive behavioral confirmation of his ability to be fluent. The content stutterer needs to reconstruct his perceptual-cognitive world and needs to test his exhibited fluency in a variety of new situations. Such an analysis gives an indication of the types of responses to be considered in therapy.

At the outset of our work we had no *a priori* criteria for the assignment of a particular stutterer to either the form or content category. Eventually, after considerable experience observing a large number of stutterers, a line of demarcation was established at a frequency of stuttering of 5 percent. Stutterers who stuttered on more than five words per each 100 uttered were placed in the form category, while those who stuttered on five words or less per 100 uttered were placed in the content category. It is interesting to note that a stutterer who seldom stutters must confirm himself as a stutterer. This is done in a variety of ways, by verbally proclaiming his fears and by participating in an intricate scheme of avoidance techniques. The form stutterer's problem is overtly manifest, while the content stutterer's problem is manifest indirectly in statements uttered by him. By simple counting we can calculate the frequency of stuttering and thus identify the form and content stutterer.

The basic rationale for considering the thematic content of a stutterer's speech as part of the problem, and therefore diagnostic or evaluative, is based on the work of the general semanticists, particularly Williams (1957). Proposed is the idea that stuttering may be maintained to a great degree by virtue of the concepts that stutterers possess. If, for example, a stutterer regards himself as the victim of unobservable entities, being the nonmalleable product of past events, and in general helpless, then therapeutic efforts should be directed to modifying these expressed beliefs. The content stutterer demonstrates an ability to be fluent but retains a strong stuttering self-concept.

CRITIQUE OF EVALUATIVE PROCEDURE

In this section we have outlined an evaluative procedure that departs significantly from the traditional ones. It can be criticized in terms of reliability and validity criteria. Do we know that the unsolicited information the stutterer reveals in an initial session is essentially the same as he will give subsequently? We do not. At the same time the traditional interviewer is faced with the same reliability problem. Unless he has built into his written and oral questionnaires some test for consistency, he is faced with the same problem. Even with the test, there is no further test for long-term consistency.

Probably the most severe criticism of our procedure would come from the operant conditioners themselves. An evaluation session usually functions as a baseline session, one in which a representativeness of behavior is observed. Representativeness can be equated with reliable here, given that under the same conditions, the stutterer would repeatedly perform in the same way. Specifically the stutterer would demonstrate no systematic changes in either the frequency of stuttering or in the distribution of thematic content statements across categories. We have addressed ourselves to this criticism within sessions and across sessions by analyzing the data from ten stutterers.

Analysis of the frequency of stuttering of eight stutterers during the first half of an evaluation session in comparison with their frequency of stuttering during the second half of that session showed no significant differences. In like manner sequential series of eight and fourteen evaluation sessions of the type we have described on two individual stutterers showed no systematic changes over time in either stuttering or content. In other words there was no significant difference between initial and later evaluation sessions for these two stutterers. With respect to the frequency of stuttering, therefore, on the basis of these data, we believe one evaluation session can yield reliable information and can therefore be utilized as baseline.

There is also a practical problem associated with extended baseline studies. We have found that stutterers will not tolerate a series of clinical interviews where in their eyes no treatment is being provided, and where in fact, no contingencies are operating.

The validity question is a source of much criticism. Does a person talking for 40 minutes produce a record that is in any way valid for diagnosing his problem and/or planning therapy for his problem? Certainly if one desires specific information, it is inadequate. The imbedded question of the value of solicited information is also involved; namely, are questions asked in a case history valid? We have seen earlier that much of the information we obtained is ignored. Little is used in a demonstrable way in planning therapy. We have therefore attempted to use a method where the stutterer, not the clinician, has the freedom. The performance in the "here and now" is the important one. The stutterer will reveal what is important to him and his problem at his own pace. And in this revelation, of course, he will incidentally demonstrate the frequency of actual stuttering episodes. The fact that a person presents himself as a stutterer in concert with a stuttering frequency of less than 5 percent provides us with a reasonable assumption that his self-percepts and self-evaluations are appropriate targets for therapy, even if such content is not manifest in great frequency in his monologue. Experience has shown that eventually during his interviews the stutterer does in fact emit utterances that reflect helplessness and victimization. This is not to say that overt stuttering at a 5 percent frequency level is not appropriate for tactics that either consequate stuttering or consequate fluency. It should be recognized that these transactions emanated from a series of clinical experiments. One such series was designed to modify content while the other was to modify overt stuttering. The 5 percent cut-off for putting some stutterers into a *content* therapy program and other stutterers into a *form* therapy program was arbitrary and dictated by the needs of the research. We have also learned that in many instances those stutterers who went through the form modification therapy later needed the content program as they achieved fluency. In some of the experiments, both types of responses were consequated as they occurred during interviews and group sessions on parallel schedules of reinforcement.

The important points to be made here are that two types of responses were observed and analyzed, *content* and *form*. If stuttering frequency was greater than 5 percent, the stutterer was put into a therapy program that was designed to manipulate the overt frequency and form of his stuttering, no matter what his content was like. If he stuttered 5 percent or less he was placed in a content program. The evaluation session was used as the vehicle for observing these responses because it would give the stutterer the greatest freedom from influence by a questioner in composing his narrative.

THERAPY

In the previous section of this chapter we described an evaluation procedure that enabled us to place stutterers into content or form categories. In this section we will present some of the therapeutic procedures we have used with stutterers in both categories. Easily recognizable and acknowledged in our applications will be the ideas of other clinicians, experimenters, and theorists.

PROGRAMS FOR THE FORM STUTTERER

Form Program One.   Our first attempts at developing for the form stutterer a therapeutic program that would attempt to modify the overt characteristics of stuttering were based on the ideas of Van Riper. Van Riper has developed a series of steps for modifying the stuttering block. Briefly the steps are: cancellation, pull-outs, and preparatory sets (Van Riper, 1963). In cancellation, the stutterer stops after each stuttered word and repeats the word in a modified way. In pulling-out, the stutterer interrupts himself during the block itself and modifies his subsequent behavior. Finally, in the preparatory set, the stutterer tries to anticipate an impending block and attempts to modify his reactions to anticipatory cues, whether phonetic, lexical, or thematic. In this manner the stutterer can generate less spasmodic speech that approaches that of the fluent individual. Our first program consisted of four steps.

Step 1: The stutterer is instructed to pause after every stuttered word and to reiterate the word, the completion of which is approved by the clinician. A reiteration of a stuttered word, even if stuttered, is accepted as a correct response if the word is reiterated before the stutterer proceeds to the next word. To separate the stuttering operant of word repetition from the program operant of reiteration, a correct response is defined as a stuttered word followed by a pause followed by an additional utterance of the word.

Step 2: This step is a refinement of the task required in Step 1. The stutterer receives approval if he reiterates a stuttered word in a prolonging pattern. The sequence of responses would be "m-m-m-man (pause) mmman."

Step 3: The stutterer receives approval in this step when he interrupts stuttering behavior while stuttering on the word and prolongs the first sound of the word being stuttered. An example of this response would be "m-m-m (Pause) mmman." The prolongation of the initial sound of the word following a whole word repetition is also considered a correct response, e.g., "not, not (pause) nnnot."

Step 4: The stutterer receives approval in this step when he prolongs the first sound of a stuttered word. An example of a correct response in this step is "mmman." A correct response is not differentiated from the stuttering operant of prolongation, and both are approved.

Schematically, the program is represented in Table 7.1. Progression

TABLE 7.1. Schematic of Form Modification Program One.

| | | Clinician's Contingent Responses | |
| | | *Positive* *reinforcement* | *Punishment* *for failure to* *complete task* |
Step	*Stutterer's Task*		
1	Pause following every stuttered word and reiterate the word.	"Good," "Fine," "That's good," "Okay," "Mm-hm," head nod, etc.	Interrupt client and repeat task instructions.
2	Reiterate stuttered word prolonging initial sound of word reiterated.	Same	Same
3	Interrupt stuttering on a word and prolong initial sound of stuttered word.	Same	Same
4	Prolong first sound of each stuttered word.	Same	Same

From Shames et al. (1969). Used by permission from the *J. of Speech and Hearing Disorders* and the authors.

through the steps of this program depended upon the stutterer's successful completion of the required step task on 90 percent of the words stuttered. When the 90 percent criterion was reached, the stutterer advanced to the next step. Base rate data were not collected before the separate steps of the program because reaching the criterion level for terminating a particular program step made the pre-therapy base rate for the next step artificial. For example, when a stutterer used a particular modification technique to alter 90 percent of his stuttered words, thus reaching the criterion level, it followed that a determination of baseline level for the next program step was contaminated by the newly acquired stuttering pattern.

A successful progression through the steps of the program systematically led to speech more closely approximating that of nonstutterers. Once the stutterer progressed to the next behavior, he was no longer reinforced for giving an earlier acquired modification response. To ensure adequate verbal output by the client, stutterer and clinician agreed upon thematic content of the discussion before the therapeutic session began. In this manner content was controlled to prevent long silent periods and to reduce the probability of emotionally loaded themes.

TABLE 7.2.   Results of Form Program One with One Stutterer.

Session	Description	Total Words	Stuttered Words	Task Completion	Percentage Task Completions for Stuttered Words	Stuttering per 100 Words
	Initial interview	2,310	314			14
	Training for Step 1					
1	Step 1	1,140	173	129	75	15
2	Step 1	1,378	105	90	86	8
3	Step 1	988	66	62	94*	7
	Training for Step 2					
4	Step 2	798	113	103	91*	14
	Training for Step 3					
5	Step 3	3,077	105	90	86	3
6	Step 3	3,178	70	59	84	2

From Shames et al. (1969). Used by permission from the *J. of Speech and Hearing Disorders* and the authors.

* 90 percent task completion criterion reached.

Table 7.2 shows the results of applying this program with a particular stutterer. Stuttering decreased from 14 stuttered words per 100 uttered to two stuttered words per 100 uttered. The decrease in stuttering was not linear. Particularly noted are the increases in stuttering frequency in the first sessions of Step 1 and Step 2, where new behavioral tasks are required of the stutterer. In running this program we were particularly impressed with the incidental decreases in stuttering frequency. The decreases were incidental because the program was designed to modify the stuttering episodes, not to eliminate them.

Form Program Two. We used the information garnered in this first form program to construct a second program of the form type. The second program was more comprehensive in terms of the number of modification steps included, and it exploited the fact that many stutterers display increases in fluency when they are ostensibly engaged in a programmed effort to modify their stuttering episodes. Table 7.3 shows Form Program Two. It can be seen that there are eight modification steps, an evaluation step (Step 1), and a final step dealing with a direct attempt to strengthen and consequate fluency and suppress stuttering. The four additional modification steps were added to "smooth out" the program. It is a cardinal rule in program construction that steps should be so designed that they are completable in a reasonable amount of time. The stutterer must have the feeling of making progress toward achieving his goal. The four additional steps take the stutterer further toward the goal of fluency. The last step in the program relates to the fact that stutterers were found to become more fluent when they were asked to engage in modification tasks. Observing this repeatedly, we decided to provide a bypass step in the program. Contingent upon 40 minutes of speech with less than 5 percent stuttering, the stutterer was advanced to Step 10 of the program. In this step we instructed the stutterer point-blank, "Talk for 40 minutes without stuttering." The rationale behind this step was that the stutterer demonstrated his ability to be increasingly fluent and we therefore sought to have this fluency maintained and increased by asking the stutterer to take responsibility for his fluent speech and verbally punishing him when he did not.

We ran this second form program with 12 adult stutterers in weekly sessions for four months. In this period of time four of the stutterers completed the program; one reached Step 10; two, Step 6; two, Step 5; and three, Step 3. We were particularly intrigued with Step 10. During earlier modification steps five stutterers' frequency of stuttering fell below 5 percent and they moved to Step 10, which consisted of continuous verbal punishment offered by the clinician contingent upon any stuttering by the stutterer. Under such a contingency four stutterers experienced reductions of stuttering to 1 percent or less. We then asked if Step 10 of

TABLE 7.3. Form Program Two.

Step	Stutterer's Task	Clinician's Contingent Response	Criterion to Move On
1	Talk for 40 minutes.*	None	More than 1,000 words More than 5 percent stuttering**
2	Do not repeat any words or phrases.	Fixed interval reinforcement for not backing up. Continuous punishment for backing up	Fewer than 1 percent repetition
3	Repeat every stuttered word	Positive reinforcement for correct responses	90 percent success
4	After every stuttered word, say the first syllable of that word 3 times and then repeat the word.	Same as Step 3	Same as Step 3
5	After every stuttered word, say the first syllable 3 times and say the word. Continue repeating the first syllable 3 times and saying the word until the word is said fluently.	Positive reinforcement when the word is said fluently	Same as Step 3
6	Same as Step 5	Positive reinforcement when the word is said fluently and on the first repetition	Same as Step 3
7	Rather than stuttering, he is to say the first syllable of a word he was going to stutter on 3 times and then say the word fluently.	Positive reinforcement for words said in the prescribed fashion	Same as Step 3
8	Same as Step 7 but he repeats the first syllable only 2 times.	Positive reinforcement*** for words said in the prescribed fashion	Same as Step 3
9	Same as Step 8 but he repeats the first syllable only 1 time.	Same as Step 8	Same as Step 3
10	No stuttering.	Positive reinforcement for intervals of fluency. Continuous verbal punishment for all stuttering****	Same as Step 3

* This task is required in all ten steps.

** If at any point in any step stuttering drops to 5 percent or less, the stutterer is moved to Step 10.

*** Positive reinforcement took the form of verbal approval: "Good job," "You're following the pattern—good."

**** Punishment took the form of verbal disapproval and rejection of responses: "You're not following instructions," "You're backing up," "No," "Stop it."

Form Program Two could be used as a complete program in itself. This question was the basis of our third form-type therapy program.

Form Program Three. Seventeen adult stutterers were enrolled as clients to test Form Program Three. The instructions given in the conditioning sessions were to "talk for 40 minutes without stuttering. Let's begin." The only contingency in effect was to have the clinician react to each stuttered word by repeating the word immediately after the stutterer stuttered on it. Pre-therapy baseline frequencies of stuttering for the 17 stutterers ranged between 4.9 percent and 50.1 percent, with a mean frequency of 15.5 percent. The instruction given to the stutterer at the outset of the first preconditioning baseline session was to *talk for 40 minutes.* In a second preconditioning session, the stutterers were given the instruction to *talk for 40 minutes without stuttering.* However, no contingent responses were made by the clinician. With this instruction in effect, it was found that during the initial part of most sessions there was a reduction in the frequency of stuttering but the reduction was transitory. Combining this information with the previous information we reported on baseline reliability, we concluded that instructions without contingencies are not sufficient to reduce stuttering. The previous information that was instrumental in this conclusion involved two additional stutterers we saw for eight and 14 sessions in which only the instruction to talk for 40 minutes was given and no contingent responses were made by the clinician. Under these conditions no systematic changes in stuttering, either increases or decreases, were observed.

After the two preconditioning baseline sessions, conditioning sessions began. The success criterion was 1 percent or less stuttering across the 40-minute period. Of the 17 stutterers seen on the program, 16 reached the 1 percent or less criterion level. The average number of 40-minute sessions required for the 16 stutterers to reach the 1 percent level was 40, with a range of eight to 59. In general there was a direct relation between the number of sessions required to reach the 1 percent level and the frequency of stuttering in the preconditioning sessions, that is, the higher the frequency of stuttering in the preconditioning sessions, the more sessions required to reach the 1 percent level.

One to three extinction sessions were conducted with each of the 16 stutterers who reached the 1 percent criterion level. The extinction sessions were characterized by the absence of contingent responses by the clinician. In the extinction sessions no stutterer's frequency of stuttering returned to 50 percent of its preconditioning level. In 11 cases, the acquired 99 percent fluency level was maintained, and in four cases fluency levels were above 90 percent.

THEMATIC CONTENT MODIFICATION PROGRAMS

It is possible that stuttering may be maintained to a great degree because of the concepts that stutterers possess, as revealed through their utterances. For example, no effective change in stuttering behavior seems feasible in therapy as long as the stutterer regards himself as being helpless and/or under the control of past events. In extensive observations of stutterers' statements, we have identified certain content themes that appear characteristic. As a result of these observations, thematic content that seemed to emerge rather consistently in the verbal responses of stutterers has been identified. By virtue of their frequency in stutterers' statements and because of their assumed relation to stuttering, two broad response classes were categorized: (1) positive statements, those utterances emitted by stutterers that were deemed beneficial to therapeutic progress because of their thematic content; and (2) negative statements, those utterances that were regarded as incompatible with recovery because of their thematic content.

Using these response categories, the thematic content modification programs were established. The general goals for the content programs were to increase the frequency of or strengthen positive (desirable) thematic responses and to decrease the rate of or weaken negative (undesirable) thematic responses during interviews. This was accomplished by instructing the clinician to "scan" the stutterer's verbalizations for statements satisfying specific definitions. To facilitate recognition of such responses, the clinician was instructed to classify them as Target Responses (TR's): a positive thematic statement was a TR+, and a negative thematic statement a TR−. The categories appear in Table 7.4. In most cases, response categories 1 through 8 are considered positive while 9 and 10 are negative. Exceptions occur. For example, Response Category 6, Negative Affect, may be positive or negative depending upon the individual stutterer and the context in which the response appears.

Thematic Content Modification Program One (TCMP1). In this program the clinician reacts favorably to TR+ statements, unfavorably to TR− responses, and engages in noncontingent responses. The clinician responds to TR+'s contingently, repeating or paraphrasing the TR, then adds a Positive Tag Line of approval, such as "I understand," "I see," "You're right," "Okay," "Good," or "mm-hm." In a like manner, he reacts to TR−'s with a repetition or paraphrase plus a Negative Tag Line of disapproval, such as "I don't understand," "No," "I don't agree," or "That's not right." These positive and negative contingent events are designed to strengthen TR+'s and to weaken TR−'s. In short, statements of approval are designed to act as positive reinforcers and statements of disapproval as mild verbal punishment. Noncontingent clinician re-

TABLE 7.4. Positive (TR+) and Negative (TR−) Thematic Content
Response Categories.

Response Category	Definition	Example
1. Concurrent Variable	Statement that reflects client's awareness or growing awareness of events or situations accompanying his stuttering or fluency	"I stutter when I'm talking on the phone," or "I don't stutter much around home."
2. Controlling Variable	Statement that reflects client's awareness or growing awareness of events controlling or causing his stuttering behavior or fluency	"Maybe I stutter because I think about how I'm going to talk before I say anything."
3. Description of Struggle Behavior	Statement that describes a client's overt motor struggle behavior when speaking	"I blink my eyes when I stutter."
4. Description of Avoidance Behavior	Statement that describes or reports a client's avoidance behavior at word, situation, and interpersonal levels	"I sometimes change words when I think I'm going to stutter."
5. Positive Affect	Statement that describes or evaluates a client's feelings or emotional state in a positive manner	"It makes me feel good not to stutter."
6. Negative Affect	Statement that describes or evaluates a client's feelings or emotional state in a negative manner	"I sometimes hate everybody in the world."
7. Contemplated Action	Statement that reports thoughts of engaging in activities or meeting situations involving speaking	"I think I'll call him on the phone tonight."
8. Completed Action	Statement that reports the completion of action involving speaking	"I finally talked to my boss today about the raise."
9. Ambiguous Amorphous Entities	Statement referring to speech or stuttering that is imprecise, vague, or nondescriptive; must contain the key words "it," "this," or "this thing"	"It occurs when I start to talk," or, "I just don't know what to do about this thing."
10. Helplessness-Victimization	Statement reflecting client's perceptions of himself as one who is helpless, incapable of acting or changing, and the victim of external events both past and present over which he has no control	"I can't get the word out," "I'm just not able to say it," "When this stuttering happens, the word gets caught and I can't get it out."

From Shames et al. (1969). Used by permission from the *J. of Speech and Hearing Disorders* and the authors.

sponses, such as "Can you tell me more?" or "Is there anything else?" are used to maintain the stutterer's verbal output and do not immediately follow the emission of a TR by the stutterer. In carrying out this program, the clinician gives no instructions to the stutterer. This program was designed primarily for those stutterers whose speech is intelligible and grammatically intact, but whose verbal output requires occasional stimulation.

Thematic Content Modification Program Two (TCMP2). The second content program, TCMP2, parallels more closely an experimental laboratory situation, and places more restrictions on the clinician's behavior. Under this program, the only critical response category is TR+, that is, no negative language responses are contingently responded to, and the clinician does not engage in noncontingent verbal behavior as he does in TCMP1. Thus in TCMP2, the clinician can sit in silence for an entire session if the stutterer fails to emit a single TR+.

In carrying out TCMP2, the clinician informs the stutterer that a therapeutic situation is being provided in which he (the stutterer) is free to speak. The stutterer is told that the therapy sessions will not be conventional conversational situations and that the clinician will sometimes respond to the stutterer's utterances and will at other times not do so. Contingent events for TR+'s are identical to those described in TCMP1.

TCMP2 was designed for those stutterers who are able to maintain an adequate level of verbal output without a great deal of clinician intervention. In addition, this program was designed to deal with stutterers whose negative thematic statement rate was relatively low. A third reason for designing TCMP2 was that we were interested in investigating the efficacy of modifying positive language only.

Thematic Content Modification Program Three (TCMP3). This program is similar to TCMP1 in that TR+'s and TR−'s are responded to contingently. But it is distinguished from TCMP1 in that noncontingent responses are not made by the clinician. TCMP3 was developed for the more verbal stutterer who may not require as frequent clinician intervention as provided by TCMP1. Contingent events for TR+'s and TR−'s are identical to those described in TCMP1. A summary of the Thematic Content Modification Programs is presented in Table 7.5.

Table 7.6 shows the results of applying the three thematic content programs with 13 adult stutterers. For the three stutterers in TCMP1, decreases in stuttering frequencies were observed. The decreases were gradual except for Stutterer 3, who showed a large initial increase. Two of the three stutterers in TCMP2 showed decreases in stuttering frequency

TABLE 7.5.   Summary of Thematic Content Modification Programs.

Program	Target Response	Clinician's Behavior
TCMP1	TR+, TR−	Positively reinforce TR+'s Punish TR−'s Intervene noncontingently to maintain client's verbal output
TCMP2	TR+	Positively reinforce TR+'s
TCMP3	TR+, TR−	Positively reinforce TR+'s Punish TR−'s

From Shames et al. (1969). Used by permission from the *J. of Speech and Hearing Disorders* and the authors.

while one showed an increase. Four of the seven stutterers in TCMP3 decreased their stuttering frequencies across therapy. Overall, nine of the stutterers displayed decreases in stuttering, ranging from a small decrement of 1 percent to a decrease of 19 percent. It is important to note that the reductions in stuttering were incidental to the therapeutic activity since this activity was focused on the thematic content of the stutterer's speech.

TABLE 7.6.   Summary of Results for Adult Stutterers on Thematic Content Modification Programs.

Stutterer	TCMP Program	Baseline Session			Final Session			Number of Sessions
		Percentage stuttering	TR+	TR−	Percentage stuttering	TR+	TR−	
1	1	4	0	0	2	1	1	18
2	1	4	8	18	2	14	13	6
3	1	14	17	47	3	30	16	18
4	2	10	0	NA	3	31	NA	14
5	2	10	22	NA	8	18	NA	12
6	2	7	6	NA	11	11	NA	7
7	3	3	0	0	2	22	7	14
8	3	23	0	2	4	15	3	18
9	3	2	14	18	3	29	8	4
10	3	6	4	0	8	10	4	8
11	3	8	8	24	3	47	0	14
12	3	8	2	8	9	15	1	12
13	3	14	0	0	8	26	1	11

NA = not applicable in this program.

In the majority of cases the number of positive thematic content statements (TR+'s) increased and correspondingly the number of negative thematic content statements (TR−'s) decreased. Thus, there is an apparent relation between the thematic content of the stutterer's speech and his overt displays of fluency and stuttering. Also, with the initial dispensing of the contingencies there were increases in stuttering above baseline.

Two findings emerged in running the content programs. First, contingent reaction to the thematic content of a stutterer's speech over a number of consecutive therapy sessions can be accompanied by concomitant reductions in the frequency of stuttering. Second, although the contingencies seem to be responsible for these incidental decreases in stuttering, we have not been able to establish a rigorous systematic relation between the distribution of TR+'s and TR−'s and stuttering frequency. Part of the problem stems from the fact that a stutterer who is making progress many times reexperiences in new situations the fears and anxieties of past situations. For example, one stutterer made marked progress in entering new situations: going to a restaurant and ordering, joining the men's club at church. In terms of situation avoidance this man was progressing, but in reporting on his behavior in these situations he uttered statements representative of helplessness and victimization. His frequency of TR−'s increased. His stuttering frequency did not. Thus in this period of therapy a direct relation between stuttering frequency and the frequency of TR−'s was nullified.

We could of course be satisfied with the favorable outcome of applying these programs and ignore the present nonsystematic relationships among therapeutic events. This prevents us from knowing more precisely about the process of amelioration. Consequently our current efforts are pointed at discovering more about the relation between thematic content and fluency.

SUMMARY

In this chapter a strategy for the evaluation of adult stutterers was presented. The goal of this particular procedure was to have the stutterer spontaneously reveal his manner of speaking and his perceptions through the vehicle of a 40-minute monologue. On the basis of listening to a number of monologues from different stutterers a classification scheme was developed. Stutterers were either form stutterers or content stutterers. Form stutterers were characterized by speech laden with hesitations, repetitions, and other overt mannerisms high in frequency and severe in nature. Content stutterers, on the other hand, exhibited speech that was essentially free from these overt behaviors. Their most salient characteristic was the possession of a percept and belief system that is compatible with a self-image of a stutterer. Such percepts and beliefs were revealed in the content of their speech samples.

Therapeutic strategies for both the form and content stutterers were developed and applied. In either case the same operant procedure was utilized. A target-response category or operant was defined. The frequency of occurrence of target responses emitted by the stutterer was counted in a preconditioning period wherein the clinician responded contingently to target responses on a specified schedule. The basic difference between the form and content programs lay with the target response. In the form program it was a motoric response while in the latter program it was one of several specified thematic content responses. The evaluation techniques provided results for the assignment of stutterers to therapeutic programs. Results from the initial application of the therapeutic programs were generally favorable. The programs provided illustrations of the direct application of operant principles to the problem of stuttering in adults.

8

....

Case
Studies

The two previous chapters contained descriptions of the therapy programs we constructed and applied. Results on groups of stuttering children and adults served by the programs were reported. In this chapter we will present in detail several case studies showing how specific stutterers progressed in therapy. Selected for presentation are two children and three adults, illustrating differing tactics with different target responses. All names used in these case studies are fictitious.

CASE ONE

Case One was a 13-year-old girl who came to the clinic with her father. Danielle was Child 9 described in the initial application of the parent-child program in Chapter Six. An evaluation was conducted according to the dictates described earlier. The father spoke with Danielle in the controlled waiting-room situation (CWS) and the clinician spoke with her in the therapy situation (TS). Percentages of stuttering in the two sessions were 2.1 percent and 1.9 percent. Danielle was accepted for therapy on the contingency that one parent would attend each therapy session with her. Her father said that he would attend, stating that he wanted to get to know his daughter better.

The father's behavior when speaking with his daughter was most vivid and easily described. He would react to his daughter's stuttering blocks by holding his ears and shaking his head while saying, "Oh no." Moreover, he seemed to be threatened by the content of his daughter's speech. At this point in time, for example, miniskirts were just beginning to become popular. Danielle talked about miniskirts and said that many girls in her parochial school "rolled up" their school uniform skirts at the waist to make them look like miniskirts. Her father's response to this was similar to his response to her stuttering block. He shook his head in a negative way saying, "Oh no, don't tell me that." Similar responses were made to other content areas reported by his daughter. Many of these topics were those of concern to young girls of her age.

Therapy began in the manner described earlier. The clinician was to relate to this child in a manner opposite to what was observed during the interactions with her father. Specifically, the clinician was open to all topics and showed interest in what Danielle had to say. Most important, the clinician avoided any nonverbal or verbal censure of Danielle's utterances. With the clinician she talked about miniskirts, pop records, boys, and so on. In addition, she talked about speech, words, and places and people, and how they make you stutter. A specific question was, "Why do [s] words make you stutter?" Reaching this point without any explicit directive was due, we believe, to the interpersonal posture taken by the clinician. The clinician was able to continue in this same posture when critical questions about speech arose. The clinician answered these questions in a number of ways. Sometimes it was by pointing out all the [s] words the child had said fluently, which seemed to stimulate more questions about stuttering. Danielle learned that you do not have to stutter on [s] words, that [s] words do not make you stutter, and that it is all right now and then to be afraid; indeed, even other people become afraid at times. All this evolved in the give and take of dyadic communication. Concomitant with these discussions were decreases in stuttering in both frequency and severity.

When stuttering frequency stabilized at 1 percent after 14 weekly sessions, Stage 2 was begun. Here the CWS was conducted before each session, but in the TS the father became a participant. Stage 2 sessions were conducted for twenty-six weeks. Across these sessions stuttering frequency continued to decrease in both the CWS and TS until stuttering was no longer part of the girl's speaking behavior. Having the father join the clinician and his child seemed most beneficial. Danielle's fluency with her father reached 100 percent and the father seemed to become much more accepting of his daughter. He was able to listen to what she had to say and separate her as a person from what she was reporting. For instance, at the outset of therapy the father thought that any description of events at school was an endorsement of these events by his daughter and promptly injected a negative evaluation. But in many cases the father's interruptive injections were premature. The child did not necessarily endorse the activity but wanted to communicate, as evidenced by subsequent remarks later in therapy when the father permitted them. For example, early in therapy Danielle reported that some musical recordings had been stolen. Her father immediately recoiled with, "Don't tell me that you've now started stealing, too." Actually Danielle was reporting an event that she had nothing to do with. It seemed that this incident as well as others was representative of her use of shock tactics to engage her father in dialogue. In later situations the father became able to make positive comparisons of his own past behavior with his daughter's. He reported events from his own youth where he had fallen short of some adult's expectations of him. There began a series of revelations from the father to the daughter and clinician during clinical sessions. These dealt mainly with the father's concern for his job. He admitted that he worried excessively about his job and that he suffered headaches as a result. In terms of advancement, the father had a series of on-time promotions in his job in a large corporation, but with each promotion the worry seemed to increase. He was concerned about whether or not he would make the next promotion. It was our impression that the father equated any admission of worry with weakness. When he was subsequently able to talk about his own fears it appeared that he did not become weak in his daughter's eyes, but human.

The father reported to us on several occasions that he thought the therapy was doing as much or more for him than for his daughter. There was one occasion when father and daughter were talking about his worry and headaches and the daughter suggested that he quit his job. The father was rather stunned and said that he could not do that, enumerating all the financial burdens that he carried. The daughter replied that the headaches were his by choice since he chose to continue to work. Following this was some banter about what the family would do and how they would live if the father quit working. The father did not quit working but the exchanges with his daughter seemed to provide gentle moments of insight, which he remarked upon repeatedly.

In the final therapy session and in reevaluation sessions eight and 12 months after therapy, the child exhibited no stuttering in either the CWS or TS. In addition, the verbal interaction between Danielle and her father changed profoundly. He was now relaxed with her. He could laugh with her, and he was able to discuss potentially sensitive topics without premature judgment and accusation.

CASE TWO

Case Two was ten-year-old John, who was accompanied to the speech evaluation session by his mother. His frequency of stuttering with his mother in CWS was 3.8 percent and with the clinician in the TS it was 4.2 percent. The mother-child interaction was characterized by the mother's constant interruptions. Moreover, there was a barrage of questions. These, in conjunction with the interruptions, gave the CWS session an appearance of an aggressive criminal interrogation. Many of the questions the mother asked she also answered. Frequently John responded to his mother with a whine of long duration. John appeared to be immature for his age. Contributing to this picture of immaturity was an [r] sound articulation problem: the boy substituted [w] for [r] in the initial position and distorted or omitted the sound in medial and final positions. John's play and attention seemed also below his chronological age. While his mother talked to him, John ran toy cars above and below the table and even on the floor, making motor noises in concert with his movements. All the while his mother questioned and answered, John paid little or no attention. The situation gave the appearance of Piaget's Collective Monologue, where two participants respond in the same situation without taking each other into account. Our goals in therapy with this child were to give him an opportunity to talk, to praise him for his ideas and thoughts, and to eliminate the whining responses by not accepting them.

Twelve sessions were held in Stage 1. Across these 12 sessions stuttering frequencies fell near the 1 percent level in both the CWS and TS, then rose to near 4 percent in the CWS, fell again in the CWS, rose a second time, and then fell and did not rise again. There were corresponding rises and falls in the TS but never above 2 percent. When stuttering frequency stabilized at less than 1 percent in the TS, Stage 2 began, and the mother was brought into the session with John and the clinician. The cyclical increases in stuttering frequencies during Stage 1 seemed related to John's attempts to converse in a manner fitting his age (sitting in a chair and attending to his conversational partner without whining). Thirteen sessions were held in Stage 2. There was a gradual decline in stuttering in both the CWS and TS sessions. In Stage 2, John acquired and maintained fluency. After he acquired fluency, we worked on the [r] problem and eliminated it. We chose to do this for a number of reasons, one of which was that it gave us an opportunity to monitor the child's newly acquired fluency. It was maintained across the duration of the articulation therapy, which lasted approximately seven months.

In treating this child we were never totally satisfied with the change in the mother's behavior. Positive changes did occur in her verbal interactions as she became less interruptive and interrogative. It was our impression, however, that the mother was generally overprotective and placed her child in a position where he would need more and more protection. For example, John was reportedly teased in school. The mother would say, "That's all right," she would take care of it. The boy apparently had no friends. The mother said she would be his friend. And indeed in the CWS when mother and son conversed this was manifest. The mother would plan what game they would play that night and where they would go for ice cream after the game. What made this overprotection so obvious was the fact that John had a younger brother who was not nearly so dependent and who had established relations with peers.

As this information and these impressions accrued over the initial therapy sessions, we thought it would be better if the father attended therapy with his son. This was never possible, although on the basis of one post-stuttering family counseling session the father did begin interacting with John, and later took him to ball games and so on.

CASE THREE

Case Three was a 42-year-old male. The content of Richard's speech during the initial interview dealt with many of the positive aspects of stuttering. He described stuttering as his "cross to bear," yet in spite of his weighty burden he had many accomplishments. With the handicaps of stuttering and only a high school education, Richard had advanced to the executive level in his division of a large industrial firm. He noted with pride and accomplishment that college graduates were under his supervision. So without a doubt he had achieved many of the vocational results that would fit the criteria of success.

Richard recounted a history of struggle with the problem of stuttering. There were many battles and some were won. He entered several public speaking classes for adults and won various awards including the "Golden Throat" award. He by his description had come a long way and the 2 percent observed frequency of stuttering in the evaluation session tended to confirm this. But there remained that final step—the move from 2 percent to 0 percent and the associated changes in his self-perception as a speaker. Here is where therapy began. Richard was placed in TCMP3, one of our content programs in which the therapist reacts with paraphrase and agreement to the stutterer's positive statements and with paraphrase and disagreement or lack of understanding to his negative statements. Content, not stuttering, was the target behavior. Topics introduced by Richard in the early sessions were primarily related to descriptions of stuttering occasions and schemes of avoidance. In Session 9 he brought up a point he considered very valuable. He had concluded that stuttering was a crutch, that it was both something that helped him and something he could blame for any failure. Like a player in Eric Berne's game (Berne, 1967, p. 92) IF WY (If it Weren't for You), by retaining some stuttering, Richard could say, "If it weren't for stuttering, I would have been flown in the company plane to the Buffalo meeting." Richard recognized that he was in the situation we call the double-bind. Stuttering was responsible for his trying harder to succeed, and therefore responsible for his success, but it was also preventing his success. After perceiving his situation, Richard decided to "go it alone," to not use stuttering as a crutch anymore. One particular overt behavior he exhibited when in a silent stuttering block was eyelid fluttering. He learned to monitor this behavior and the situations in which it occurred. He reported much success in controlling eyelid fluttering and in "going it alone."

A second cognitive breakthrough occurred near the end of therapy. Richard said he had finally had a long talk with his wife about stuttering. She told him that when she married him she did not think she would be married to a stutterer all her life. She said it was all right to be fluent. This release seemed very important to Richard; it allowed him to become the man he wanted to be.

As we saw the importance of interpersonal dynamics in parent-child dyads, we can see the importance of such dynamics here. Richard's wife accepted him and his stuttering when she married him and lived with his struggles against the "stuttering beast" throughout the years. His wife accepted him when others apparently did not. Would he betray her now by becoming fluent? His fluency would disrupt an equilibrium that included stuttering. The assurance from his wife that it was all right to be fluent seemed to be the key to this man's efforts in acquiring fluency. He became fluent and remained so during three subsequent reevaluations 18 months after therapy. Overall there was a total of 15 therapy sessions.

This case illustrates the difficulty of using raw frequencies of positive and negative thematic content responses. As we reported, there were two prominent insights verbalized by the man. The first was that he now saw stuttering as a crutch, and the second was that he feared fluency would not be "fair" to his wife: These two statements seemed to carry more weight in terms of his recovery than any of the other positive content statements that Richard uttered. However, in terms of a raw count of responses they would be equal to any other pair of statements. It is probably because of this disparity between the impacts of various content statements in terms of recovery that we were not able to establish a systematic relation between thematic content and frequency of stuttering, except at global levels.

CASE FOUR

Case Four was a 23-year-old male. During the initial evaluation session Robert stuttered on 15.7 percent of his words. He was assigned to Form Program Three. The contingency in this program was continuous verbal punishment, contingent on each occurrence of stuttering. We sometimes refer to Robert's therapy as our exercise in tenacity. There were 72 conditioning sessions, five days a week, for 15 weeks. Each session was 40 minutes. There was a generally progressive rise in stuttering frequency, reaching a zenith in Session 46, with a stuttering frequency of 56 percent. Thereafter stuttering frequency dropped gradually until it fell below 1 percent in the final sessions. Periodically, thereafter, ten extinction sessions were run during which Robert maintained a fluency level in excess of 99 percent. When Robert demonstrated that he was able to maintain the 99 percent fluency level he was placed in a group of fluent stutterers, i.e., fluent in therapy but not totally fluent outside therapy.

In this group, discussions were related primarily to taking the fluency acquired in the clinic to outside situations. The young man began to make some life-style changes while in the group. He quit his job as a shipping and warehouse employee, and entered college with his veteran's benefits. On a recent informal office visit Robert reported that graduation was near, and that he still stutters now and then but that he now knows why he stutters and can stop stuttering and continue speaking without stuttering. The purpose of his visit was to announce that he had formed a group of stutterers and exstutterers. The group was to be a nonprofessional, nonprofit aggregate similar to the many ad hoc groups that form around a particular problem or issue.

CASE FIVE*

Case Five was a 47-year-old, unmarried female from a rural, disadvantaged background. Freida's father died when she was five, leaving her mother and siblings to maintain the farm. Gradually the siblings

* Much of the material presented here is from Egolf et al. (1971). Used by permission from the *J. Speech and Hearing Disorders* and the authors.

left home, leaving her to care for her mother until the mother's death. Freida left school in the eighth grade and became employed as a printing machine operator. Following her mother's death, she lived with her sister's family in the city.

Freida stuttered on 3.7 percent of her words during the initial interview. In this session her stuttering was severe. Severity was measured on a three-point scale, where a rating of one meant mild repetition or prolongation behavior with no struggle; a rating of two referred to repetition or prolongation behavior with struggle; and a rating of three referred to repetition and prolongation accompanied by extreme struggle behavior and long duration of the episode. Freida had a Severity Rating of three. Word output in the session was in slight excess of 2,400 words. In general, Freida's stuttering was characterized by blocking and sound, syllable, and word repetition. This behavior was accompanied by loss of eye contact, facial tremors, breath holding, and hand wringing.

Throughout the initial interview, she appeared depressed, speaking in a low volume with her head lowered. She presented a naive picture of herself and her stuttering. She continually referred to herself as "little me" and to "normal" people as "lucky," saying, "How do they do it (talk without stuttering)?" She referred to stuttering as her "cross to bear," as something that "just happened to her," as "it," and her "handicap." "Normal" people never paused or repeated when talking; they never made social "errors" such as spilling their coffee.

Freida reported having had speech therapy many years ago, but apparently this had not led to any reduction in the severity or frequency of her stuttering, nor to any insight into her speech problem. At the time of the initial interview, Freida reported avoiding many situations in which she might be required to converse. Her only active attempt to control her stuttering was by breathing deeply. In addition to her stuttering problem, Freida reported that her hand trembled when writing in the presence of others and when holding a cup of coffee. We observed this tremor when she was signing a release form during the first session.

Stage 1 was designed to involve Freida in the therapeutic process. As noted above, she did not look at the clinician during the initial interview. This, combined with the fact that she talked about events in her remote past as though they were current, revealed feelings of victimization and helplessness, and behavior that was suggestive of depression and withdrawal. We decided that the initial therapeutic strategy should be designed to ensure that Freida was interacting with the clinician. To satisfy this strategy, in Stage 1 Freida was instructed to talk for 40 minutes and to look at the clinician when talking. It was decided that Stage 1 would be terminated when the frequency of loss of eye contact fell below 1 percent of the number of total words that she uttered.

The instructions to the clinician in Stage 1 were to make two types of responses. The first response was labeled the "look-at-me" response. Whenever the client was talking and not looking at the clinician, the clinician would say, "Look at me." The second type of response was labeled a "verbal lubricant." A verbal lubricant is a verbal response by the clinician designed to stimulate verbal output without interpreting or biasing the content of the client's speech. Some examples of verbal lubricants are "Is there anything else?" and "Can you tell me more?"

Four sessions were held in Stage 1. During the first session the client lost eye contact 61 times; during the second, 38 times; the third, 17 times; and the fourth, 13 times. The criterion for the termination of Stage 1 was reached in Session 4. Stuttering frequency during these four sessions averaged 3.5 percent. The stuttering severity rating remained high, averaging 2.79 on a three-point scale. Word output averaged 1,503.5 words per session.

Thus, at the end of Stage 1, Freida was able to maintain eye contact, showed a slight decrease in stuttering frequency, and maintained verbal output. Her initial gains were such that she not only seemed a good candidate for therapy, but gave a good prognosis as well.

In Stage 2 of therapy, Freida was placed on TCMP3 (Thematic Content Modification Program Three). In this program, the stutterer is instructed to talk for 40 minutes. The instructions to the clinician are to react with verbal approval to any positive thematic statement the stutterer utters, and with verbal disapproval to any negative thematic statement. Positive statements are those utterances deemed beneficial to therapeutic progress because of their thematic content; negative statements are those regarded as incompatible with recovery because of their thematic content. The process of verbal approval involves the clinician's paraphrasing the stutterer's positive statement and adding a tag line such as "I agree" or "I think that's good." Verbal disapproval, on the other hand, involves the paraphrase of the negative statement followed by a tag line such as "I don't understand" or "I don't agree with that."

The theoretical basis for Stage 2 was Johnson's semantic theory of stuttering (Johnson, 1958), particularly as amplified by Williams (1957). Williams postulated that much of the difficulty experienced by stutterers arises from the way they think about stuttering and their reactions to their thoughts. For example, if the stutterer regards stuttering as some vague, indefinable happening, he is unable to analyze his own behavior, and such analysis is prerequisite to making specific behavioral changes.

Freida seemed to be a good candidate for the program since she viewed her stuttering as some affliction visited upon her, and as something she ought to bear bravely since other people had greater burdens than she.

Twenty-four sessions were held in Stage 2 during which stuttering frequency and severity decreased. Stuttering frequency, for example, averaged 3.2 percent, and stuttering severity averaged 2.4 percent. There were an average of 15.2 positive thematic statements and 12.7 negative content statements per session during Stage 2. Word output averaged 1,975.6 words per session. Interpretation of the content and frequency of these statements showed that Freida was able, at the end of Stage 2, to describe reliably her stuttering in terms of the things which she did when she talked. These descriptions accounted for the majority of her positive statements. Freida still felt "helpless" about making any changes in her behavior outside the clinic. The interpretation of "helpless" was made from her many statements beginning with "I can't." Such statements made up the bulk of her negative statements in Stage 2.

The helplessness inferred from statements in Stage 2 seemed to stem from Freida's fear that a catastrophe would occur if she stuttered or made a faux pas, such as spilling coffee in public. This fear was so pervasive that she seemed completely unaware of other people's behavior, even when she was in their presence. With these impressions in mind, it was decided to construct therapy for Stage 3 in such a way that (1) almost any behavior would be tolerated except avoidance behavior, and (2) Freida would be forced to observe the behavior of other people. As a consequence, three rules were given to her.

1. Talk whenever you want to or whenever you have the opportunity.
2. Do not care whether or not you stutter (operationally this meant keep on talking even if you stutter).
3. When you are in doubt about anything you have done, just look around and see what most people do in the same situation.

The theoretical bases for Stage 3 are contained in Sheehan's approach-avoidance theory and in Johnson's semantic theory. Rules 1 and 2 were suggested by Sheehan's theory (1958b). Deducible from this theory is that stuttering frequency will decrease if the avoidance drive is decreased. Therefore, the first two rules were designed to eliminate all tendencies to avoid. Rule 3 was suggested by Johnson's idea that the stutterer must acquire a thoroughgoing tolerance for normal behavior, which contains speech nonfluencies, hesitations, revisions, mistakes, and emotional reactions. This seemed especially appropriate for Freida since her views about normal people were highly unrealistic.

In introducing the program for Stage 3, the clinician presented the three rules to Freida. At the beginning of each subsequent session, Freida was asked to review the rules and then tell how she was doing. Session length remained 40 minutes. The clinician was instructed to approve verbally any statement that indicated Freida was following the rules and to disapprove verbally any statement that indicated she was not following the rules. A major difference between Stage 2 and Stage 3 was that reports of avoidance behavior were verbally approved in Stage 2 because they showed that the client could successfully identify and describe her behavior, but were not approved in Stage 3 because they were in violation of the rules, specifically Rules 1 and 2.

Some typical exchanges in Stage 3 were as follows:

Freida:	Well, I just couldn't ask the elevator operator for 12 so I walked up from ten.
Clinician:	What are you supposed to do?
Freida:	I'm supposed to talk.
Clinician:	Did you do that?
Freida:	No.
Clinician:	Why didn't you do that?
Freida:	I was afraid I was going to stutter.
Clinician:	What do your rules tell you about that?
Freida:	Talk and don't care if you stutter.
Clinician:	That's right. You see you didn't follow the rules. That's why you were in trouble.
Freida:	I don't order coffee because I'm afraid I'll spill it.
Clinician:	What do most people do when they spill coffee?
Freida:	They just keep right on going.
Clinician:	That's right, they just keep right on going.

Fifteen sessions were held in Stage 3. During these sessions, stuttering frequency and severity decreased. For the 15 sessions the average frequency was 2.11 percent and the average severity rating, 1.99 percent. Word output averaged 1,610.4 words per session. The average number of positive responses and negative responses was 8.8 and 8.5.

Freida was discharged after 15 sessions in Stage 3. Discharge was based upon mutual agreement of the clinician and the stutterer. Freida's request for discharge appeared to be justified, because she seemed to be asking for responsibility and independence. Although the changes in frequency and severity of stuttering were small, they were, nevertheless, in the desired direction and had been maintained, giving further merit to her request. In addition, Freida reported an incident that seemed to be indicative of success, as well as very encouraging to her. The incident was nonvocal and occurred in an "expensive" restaurant. Freida dropped her fork and "just asked the waiter for another one." The incident, trivial to most people, was a bench mark in this woman's recovery. At the time of discharge, arrangements were made for a reevaluation in six months.

The first reevaluation showed that Freida had not only maintained her therapeutic gains, but also had improved further. Her stuttering frequency was 1.22 percent, her severity rating was 1.23, and she uttered 2,618 words. She reported many more speaking contacts and reported making plans to complete high school. A second reevaluation was scheduled for six months hence, and was conducted by a second person. On this occasion Freida uttered 4,496 words and did not stutter. She reported the attainment of two important life goals: the completion of her high school education and the passing of a driver's test. In addition, she reported many new activities—traveling to Florida, dating, and so on. Freida was congratulated and told to call us now and then, just to keep in touch.

This stutterer progressed through three individualized stages of therapy with subsequent changes in her behavior. Although the stages did not adhere strictly to all the principles of operant conditioning (base rate data and extinction data), the procedures were operant to the extent that contingent responses by the clinician were employed in every session.

During therapy, Freida's stuttering decreased both in frequency and severity so that she was completely free of stuttering during the last reevaluation. In addition, there were significant changes in her interpersonal relations and personal development.

It is important to note that we were working with an extremely naive person, rather than someone who had experienced years of therapy for stuttering. To a degree, our program was adapted to this stutterer's needs, not only to help her acquire insight into her problem, but also to provide her with guidelines to follow when she encountered situations she had consistently avoided and therefore never experienced. Therapy focused primarily on behavior and attitudes related to stuttering. Attempts to modify directly the overt manifestations of stuttering were not made. However, a form of behavior closely related to overt stuttering, eye contact, was dealt with in Stage 1. Working on eye contact served two purposes for this stutterer. She demonstrated her ability to change; and she was able to observe the listener's reaction to her speech and relate directly to another person in a speaking situation.

Throughout Stages 2 and 3, it became apparent that the raw frequency of positive and negative content statements was not a critical factor in assessing her progress. However, there was a sustained decrease in the frequency and severity of stuttering events. During Stage 2, Freida explored her behavior in both positive and negative terms. For example, she learned to talk about stuttering as something she did, and not as her handicap. She also described her inability to handle speaking situations. This accounts for the slight decrease in positive content statements during the latter part of Stage 2. A more experienced stutterer might have increased positive thematic statements by reporting behavior and making positive thematic statements about stuttering based on other therapy experiences.

During Stage 3, Freida actively employed the guidelines we gave her, both in the session and in other speaking situations. She had to be involved. Although stuttering continued to decrease in frequency and severity, no systematic change was observed in the frequency of positive and negative thematic responses. We believe that this was due largely to Freida's reporting her failures to follow the guidelines and expressing her feelings about how much more she needed to accomplish. This was attested to by the fact that during Stage 3 she formulated and set about reaching goals in other aspects of her life. She actively pursued and eventually acquired a high school diploma. She obtained a driver's license. She changed her social patterns to the extent that she entered into group social activities with her boyfriend.

We believe the observations made in Freida's case have implications for work with stutterers who have had little or no previous therapy. The clinician may not have to work directly on modifying overt stuttering behavior for the stutterer to become fluent. Talking about stuttering and achieving personal insight into the problem does not guarantee fluency. To become comfortably fluent the stutterer appears to benefit if he has guidelines to use in evaluating his speech, the speaking situation, and the reactions of others in his environment.

Finally, Freida's case demonstrates the possibilities in designing therapy programs. Long-standing theories need not be abandoned in order to adopt operant procedures. If a stutterer presents a picture that is best described by a particular theory, then the behaviors that theory deems critical can be manipulated by the employment of operant procedures.

SUMMARY

In this chapter, and indeed in this part, we have reported on the application of a variety of therapeutic strategies and techniques. We anticipate that clinicians may have a number of questions as they consider the use of some of these techniques in their professional activities with stutterers. From our own experience in orally describing our procedures these questions most often begin with, "What do you do if . . ." To answer questions of this nature it may be helpful to list some of the things that can happen in therapy: the stutterer can increase his frequency of stuttering; he can remain silent; he can withdraw or stop coming to therapy; he can bait the clinician or force the clinician to deviate from his program; he can question the qualifications of the clinician and the validity of the therapeutic effort; and he can become fluent in the therapy session but continue to stutter in other situations. Such behaviors on the part of the stutterer do not, of course, fit the idealized curve of decreased frequencies of stuttering across sequential therapeutic sessions. How should the clinician respond to these disruptions occurring on the way to the therapeutic goal of having the stutterer become comfortably fluent. We shall look at these problems both in general and specific terms.

The overall recommendation for preventing these problems as much as possible is preparation. A clinician should face his client with a plan or program of therapy that has been carefully prepared and is suited to the client's needs. Preparation involves searching his history as a clinician in combination with searching the available literature on stuttering therapy. A plan of therapy should contain the reasons for its potential success. One general problem that remains is that of tenacity. How tenacious should a clinician be in applying a particular program? Like the fisherman who feels that with just one more cast the prize will be caught, so the clinician feels that with just one more session a therapeutic milestone will be successfully reached. Our own Case Study Four is an example where such thinking was successful. In therapy the man's stuttering rose in frequency to a high point in Session 46, and thereafter it continually decreased. We would predict that most clinicians would be less patient than were we, and, quite possibly another program would have achieved similar decrements in stuttering frequency in less time and without the initial increase. There are no simple and valid rules for determining the point at which a therapeutic strategy should be abandoned or modified. Consulting the available literature is helpful. For example, if DAF is used to bring about fluency, fluency should occur in a relatively short period of time. Other approaches that tie fluency reduction to overall attitude changes may predictably take longer. Consulting one's clinical history is also helpful. There is the yet-to-be-fully-described clinical hunch or impression that is many times valid. Clinicians sometimes just seem to know whether favorable results will be forthcoming on the basis of their past clinical experiences. Overall, we believe that evaluation points should be incorporated into the therapy plan to aid in any subsequent decision about the continuation or termination of a therapeutic strategy.

Many of the problems that arise in therapy can be prevented or attenuated by immediately establishing and communicating to the client the rules of therapy. For example, we instructed our clients that even though the therapeutic arrangement looked like a typical conversational arrangement (clinician and client seated together in a room), it indeed was more than that. We established for ourselves certain rules to be operative for 40 minutes and we followed our rules. We were not cold and callous. We talked to our clients before and after the 40-minute session and even discussed their performance in the session. But during the session the rules were followed. In addition, we established rules about attendance. After three unannounced absences the client's therapy time was reassigned. We believe that informing the client about such procedures communicates to him our seriousness about the therapeutic endeavor, forces a commitment from him, and makes the execution of therapy easier.

For example, one client began his 40-minute session by saying that he was getting nowhere, and that he would quit and look for another "school" of therapy. Such content from a stutterer can be threatening and disheartening to a clinician. It can bait him into departing from his program and engaging in a conversation about the stutterer's threatened withdrawal. The clinician in this case did not depart but followed the prescribed therapy program. At the end of 40 minutes the clinician noted that the client was fluent when he talked about quitting therapy. The reaction was not to the client's threat to quit but to the fluency emitted when he was on this topic.

In similar ways stutterers can test the limits with clinicians by remaining silent, introducing loaded content themes, and questioning the clinician's qualifications. Silence can be very threatening to both clinician and client. At the same time, it should not trigger any unplanned response. At the end of 40 minutes of silence the clinician might point out to the client that nothing was said in the session and that for progress to occur the client would have to begin to talk. (In actuality we have never had a client remain totally silent for 40 minutes, although one client did display silent periods of up to 20 minutes.) The client comes to learn that there is a performance time and a time to talk about the performance time. While we have no comparative statistics available, we believe that such structure sharply reduces the problems caused by happenings we have not anticipated.

What about the stutterer who becomes fluent in therapy but in no other situation? In part this problem is a creation of our professional pessimism. We have been so preoccupied with having the stutterer achieve fluent speech patterns that we have failed to plan in any way for carryover. Our present view is that this planning should begin early in therapy and we comment elsewhere in this regard. For the stutterer who has achieved fluent speech but who at the same time exhibits no carryover of that fluency, a revision in the therapy program is required. The therapy is out of phase. We would plan a carryover program for him that would require him to meet a series of speaking goals outside the therapy situation.

Perhaps, the most important point in this discussion is the realization that often there are profound differences between what we expect will occur as a result of our plans and tactics and what in fact does occur. The stutterer has not read the book, and his responses to a set of tactics and the clinician's consequent reactions to his responses may not be a mirror of the blueprint. We should be prepared for these actualities and departures. But we must also survive them. Our particular survival kit is to turn to the principles that underlie the tactics. While we may abandon a particular clinical strategy, it is our application of the underlying principles that will generate other, hopefully effective, strategies for the individualized reactions of stutterers to their therapy program.

III

NEW
DIRECTIONS
AND
CONSIDERATIONS

9

....

Introduction
to Part III

The principles of operant conditioning are conceptualizations about behavior in general, and not specifically about stuttering behavior. As a result they may profitably be applied to any observable behavior. As such, operant principles may have an accommodating property relative to traditional theories of stuttering. This section of the book deals with this accommodating property by reviewing specific applications to the Travis, Sheehan, Johnson, and Van Riper views of stuttering. The applications demonstrate some of the possible ways that operant principles can render these views more descriptive, operational, and, therefore, more clinically functional.

There is also a generative aspect to the operant model. The various ways operant conditioning has generated new information, has generated its own clinical technology, or has made use of operant-based information that has been applied to other clinical problems is also reviewed. This generative property provides a view of newer clinical potentials as well as an awareness of issues in therapy that may need to be made more prominent and explicit.

VARIABLES AFFECTING
CLINICAL TACTICS

The principles of operant conditioning, which state that behavior can be shaped, changed, maintained, strengthened, and weakened by its contingent consequence, may be characterized as atheoretical. By not being bound to any particular theoretical point of view about stuttering, these principles enjoy a freedom of application to a number of points of view, as long as the rules inherent in the principles are satisfied.

During therapy one may observe or arrange for the occurrence of certain antecedent and contingent consequent events around an observable target response that may emanate from any theory about the problem of stuttering. Likewise, these theories may also provide information about the nature and form of antecedent and consequent events that may control the occurrence of stuttering.

Most typically, when these operant principles have been applied to the clinical management of stuttering, the target response has been the stutterer's overt motor speech act. This attention to the overt speech act has taken several different directions. There have been attempts to strengthen already existing fluency, to shape slow rates of speech to fluency, to modify the form of stuttering, and to suppress stuttering. Yet, as clinicians, we know that there is more to a human speaker than his speaking machinery, and we also know that there is more to the problem of stuttering than its overt frequency of occurrence. A number of other classes of responses are pertinent to therapy for stuttering and may require intervention. These would include the stutterer's beliefs about himself, his feelings and emotions, his sense of independence and self-responsibility, and his social behavior. Each of these types of responses has received some attention within the operant framework for their pertinence to the total stuttering problem.

Attention has also been given to exploring the tactical therapeutic value of employing different forms of contingent clinician behavior. Such processes as positive reinforcement, negative reinforcement, and punishment have been studied for their clinical viability. These events have taken the form of verbal approval, smiling, money, points, acceptance, and understanding as positive reinforcers. Verbal disapproval, rejection, shock, DAF, noise, and counting instances of stuttering have been studied as contingent suppressive stimuli.

More recently, increased formalized attention has been given to programming the occasions for target responses and their consequation, as part of the clinical carryover process. The research on each of these three elements of the operant paradigm (occasions, classes of responses, and forms of contingent consequences) illustrates the diversity of interest, the broad-based need for information, and the numerous possibilities for developing and organizing a system of clinical tactics that are associated with an operant approach to therapy for stuttering. It also brings into sharper focus the possible applications of operant methodology to current and past theoretical positions about stuttering. Although the set of principles may be atheoretical (content-free), they can generate a number of clinical tactics and paradigms that may be applicable to theories of stuttering which heretofore were not conceptualized within their purview. Each of these clinical issues will be discussed in this part, as well as others where gaps in our information currently exist.

It is the purpose of Part Three to discuss and to illustrate how the principles of operant conditioning can both accommodate traditional theory and tactics and generate a number of new clinical tactics within its framework.

Being atheoretical, these principles appear to have a broad scope of application. Tactics can range over a number of types of target responses, from the overt motor speech acts of the stutterer to his most private feelings.

We will try to probe systematically the numerous possibilities for arranging therapeutic encounters: the various occasions; the different target responses; the forms and nature of the consequences; the sources of the consequences; the scheduling of the paradigm; and the stutterers' characteristics that have been suggested as variables in the therapeutic process. Sorting these issues into viable clinical tactics is a job that is well under way, but not yet completed. The principles of operant conditioning provide a rigorous and systematic way of asking questions about these issues in our work, because operant conditioning is a cautious and documented approach to the problem.

10

....

The Generative
and Accommodating Nature
of Operant Conditioning

ATTITUDES, BELIEFS, AND FEELINGS

One of the primary values of the operant framework of the various theoretical positions about stuttering is that in the statements of the relations among events viewed as basic to the nature of stuttering, we can identify classes of pertinent target behavior. Many of these responses may be in the realm of what Homme refers to as coverants (Homme, 1965). According to Homme, a coverant is a covert operant event that may function in such personal activities as thinking, creating, and imagining. These behaviors are acquired in accordance with the same principles that explain the acquisition of overt behaviors. We note that traditional theoretical views of stuttering contain statements of relations among pertinent events, some of which are based on observation and others which are inferential and hypothetical. A theory cannot be verified without behavioral observation. It is this verification by behavior observation that provides the opportunity for applying operant tactics and principles to that theoretical view of the problem of stuttering. This perception of the usefulness of traditional stuttering theory in concert with the concept of the coverant expands the possibilities for applying operant conditioning to stuttering. It is possible to deal with such constructs and private events as anxiety, conflict, feelings, attitudes, and anticipations, as long as they are translated into observable events that may be targeted for appropriate consequation.

Some of the case studies and tactics described in earlier portions of this book are examples of operant approaches which focused on target responses other than the motor speech act.

The content modification programs in which an interviewer provided approval for desirable content themes (i.e., utterances reflecting behavioral description, insight statements and evaluations, communicative and social approach behavior, and contemplated and completed action), and disapproval for undesirable content themes (i.e., utterances reflecting helplessness, victimization, the operation of ambiguous, amorphous entities) was viewed as an application of operant conditioning tactics to the semantic theory of stuttering (Shames et al., 1969). It was felt that what stutterers said out loud about themselves reflected what they believed and felt about themselves, and that these beliefs influenced their social behavior and talking behavior (stuttered and fluent). If such relations operate between what a stutterer believes about himself and how he behaves relative to these beliefs, then a legitimate therapeutic tactic is to modify that belief system (by consequating overt utterances that reflect beliefs) in an effort to affect desirable changes in social and talking behavior. The research described in Chapters Seven and Eight did in fact support these tactics and demonstrated that the content of utterances could be modified through operant tactics. It also demonstrated that these changes were associated with changes in stuttering. Such content modification programs can be designed to meet the special needs of specific stutterers.

In one such project it was felt that a stutterer who had reached a plateau in his progress in symptom management therapy was having serious difficulties in expressing hostility and aggression (Honeygosky, 1966). This view of stuttering is a direct outgrowth of the Travis theory of stuttering, which relates to the stutterer's unspeakable feelings (Travis, 1957). An examination of this stutterer's case history and of his therapy interviews revealed that he expressed very little affect of any kind, positive or negative. A clinical conditioning program was designed involving a series of eleven 50-minute interviews on a twice-a-week basis. The interviewer was instructed to ask ten key questions per interview (approximately every five minutes), which were designed to evoke an affective utterance (positive or negative). If the stutterer emitted an affective utterance on these occasions, the interviewer verbally responded with approval, acceptance, and understanding. If an affective utterance was not emitted, the interviewer withheld his verbal approval and acceptance. In his base operant level interview, this stutterer emitted one affective response, while in his final clinical session, he emitted 47 negative affective responses. His stuttering frequency decreased from four stutters per minute in his first interview to two stutters per minute in Session 11. As a short-term project, it demonstrated several things. One was that operant tactics could be applied to the Travis theory of stuttering, insofar as overt and manifest content of utterances reflect "unspeakable feelings." Second, this project demonstrated that it was possible to change what stutterers say out loud about themselves and about their relations with people, within the content of a clinical interview, in accordance with descriptive and operational principles of conditioning. Third, it demonstrated that changes in such content were associated with decrements in stuttering.

In a similar project with an adult male stutterer, a different type of content was targeted for consequation. The stutterer was not making reasonable progress in a symptom management program and it was decided that he was having difficulty in making decisions and in establishing general goals for himself, and specific goals regarding his stuttering problem and his therapy. Given the assumption of a semantic relation between our attitudes and beliefs and how we behave relative to these beliefs, a content modification program during a series of clinical interviews was designed (Johnson, 1966; Shames, 1969). The target responses for positive reinforcement were statements reflecting the description and establishment of goals and statements reflecting independent decision-making. Eighteen 50-minute interviews were held. During each interview, the interviewer asked eight to ten questions designed to evoke the target content responses. Any time the stutterer emitted a target response to a key question, he received approval and acceptance from the interviewer. If a target response were not emitted when a key question was asked, the interviewer verbally responded with disapproval and rejection.

In the stutterer's base rate session, he emitted four target responses. He also emitted four inappropriate responses in this session. In his last three conditioning sessions, he averaged approximately 31 target responses per interview (29, 31, and 32 responses in Sessions 16, 17, and 18). The frequency of his disapproved responses during these last three interviews were 4, 3, and 2, or an average of 2+ per interview.

Associated with these content changes were changes in speech repetition behavior. In the base rate session he repeated 12 times per minute. This dropped to two per minute in the final session.

Case 5, presented in Chapter Eight, is still another illustration of tactics that focused on the stutterer's feelings and beliefs. Freida went through a content modification program during 24 clinical interviews. Desirable content increased and undesirable content decreased. Also, the frequency and severity of her stuttering decreased. However, there were still residual feelings of helplessness reflected in her overt utterances in interviews. At this point, the stutterer was given three instructions based in part on the approach-avoidance theory of Sheehan (1958b) and on the semantogenic theory of Johnson (1958). Fifteen additional clinical interviews were held that focused on how well the stutterer implemented these instructions. As a result, desirable content increased further and stuttering frequency and severity decreased.

During follow-up studies and interviews the client did not stutter and she was taking significant steps in pursuing important social and occupational goals.

Each of these operant-based projects, which attempted to modify the manifest content of utterances emitted by stutterers during clinical interviews, was based on the assumption that manifest thematic content was related to the beliefs and feelings of the stutterer. It was felt that the stutterer acted on these beliefs. Therefore, the desirable changes in overt stuttering that were associated with change in manifest thematic content of utterances appeared to validate that assumption. However, it is possible that changes in stuttering can occur quite independently of changes in beliefs. At one time or another, we have all observed stutterers who have achieved total fluency in their speech and yet still believed that they were stutterers. Although the stutterer's speech behavior may interact with his beliefs and feelings about himself, each may constitute separate response classes, requiring separate and differing clinical tactics.

Just as the problem of stuttering may be more complicated than its overt frequency of occurrence, the beliefs and feelings of the stutterer appear to be much more complicated than the overt manifest thematic content of his utterances. There are private dimensions to beliefs and feelings that are not often made public and observable. Clinicians have become alert to looking for clues to these private events. We infer latent content, interpret the symbolism of manifest content, observe posture and eye contact, scan the entire array of verbal and nonverbal behaviors presented to us, in an effort to read the stutterer's moods, feelings, and internal agitation. Far too often these clues are too obscure to be recognized and clinicians have to resort to the concepts of a particular theory, and, by definition and assumption, attribute a set of feelings to a stutterer (i.e., by definition in some theories stutterers are anxious, afraid, in conflict, anticipate, and dread talking etc.). Assuming that the emotions of the stutterer are pertinent and significant to his therapy, then judgments about these emotions must be made with minimal error. Obviously, changing the manifest content of utterances is not the same as changing the feelings of the stutterer. The manifest content is concerned with the verbal, cognitive, and intellectual processes of the stutterer. His feelings may be based on internal, autonomic, physiological arousal, and excitement (Miller, 1969). Both are important to the way the stutterer views himself, thinks about himself, and feels about himself and his world.

Recent research from the fields of experimental psychology and psychosomatic medicine, dealing with biofeedback techniques, appears to have direct application to the issue of the stutterer's beliefs and feelings, and may provide a system for getting at the more private side of stuttering.

Biofeedback is a process of making public and observable, indicators of internal body activity. Patients learn to regulate these external indicators of internal activity by attaching contingent consequences to the patient's performance. For example, certain muscle activity can be represented on an EMG recorder by the movement of a pointer on a dial, or heart rate and blood pressure can be shown by visual feedback of the movement of a pen on a polygraph. The patient is instructed to keep the pen or the pointer within some predesignated range of movement. By attaching external consequences to the regulation of these indicators of internal activity, patients have learned to slow their pulse rate, and heartbeat, to lower their blood pressure, and to sustain stable GSR patterns. Kimmel (1967), Katkin and Murray (1968), and Miller (1969) have presented overviews of this research, which demonstrated instrumental control over visceral responses. Those responses that have been systematically studied have included systolic blood pressure, heart rate, alpha EEG rhythms, and GSR. These operant modifications of autonomic activity have been correlated to paradigms of positive reinforcement and punishment, as well as to specific occasions such as self-induced thoughts and mental states. Miller and DiCara (1967), Shapiro and Crider (1967), Miller (1969), Fetz and Smith (1969), Tursky and Shapiro (1969), Shapiro et al. (1970), Nowliss and Kamiya (1970), Schwartz (1970), and Finley (1971) have shown that these many different types of visceral responses, which are often related to states of excitement and emotionalism, can be controlled through biofeedback and operant conditioning procedures.

We have just begun to conceptualize the value and application of biofeedback procedures to stuttering. Gray and England (1968) demonstrated that it was possible to manipulate stutterers' electro-skin conductance responses independent of changes in stuttering behavior. Their project was not conceptualized within the biofeedback procedure, but rather was part of a desensitization and deconditioning procedure. Their interpretation of the results was that anxiety (as measured by electro-skin conductance) could be manipulated as a response independent of stuttering. It is an early example of a method for dealing with the internal physiological activity that may reflect the stutterer's emotionality. Treon et al. (1972) reported that lowered stuttering rates were associated with self-regulated monitoring of low amplitude GSR patterns. Higher stuttering rates were associated with self-regulated monitoring of high amplitude GSR patterns. In this instance, the stutterer's GSR pattern was manipulated to study the effects on stuttering.

Reed and Lingwall (1973) approached the problem from the opposite direction. They manipulated stuttering and determined the effects on the stutterer's GSR pattern. They reported that in some stutterers a consistent change in GSR activity was observed in association with contingent aversive stimulation for instances of stuttering. However, these changes in GSR, as a function of suppressing stuttering, were not in the same direction for all stutterers in the study. Although these two studies have correlated GSR to the stutterer's speech act, such information about internal activity does not necessarily have to be limited to that class of the stutterer's responses. It was mentioned earlier that the stutterer's beliefs and feelings could be dimensionalized in terms of the manifest content of his utterances and by indicators of internal autonomic activity (emotional excitement). It is suggested here that the various things the stutterer talks about during interviews, which on the surface appear to deal with his beliefs and feelings, may be associated with different states of internal excitement and emotion. We may wish to consider clinical tactics that attach certain contingent consequences to content supported by indicators of internal excitement, and different consequences to content associated with relative calm. One type of content may have a great deal of emotional clout to it and may be getting close to the stutterer's feelings and beliefs, while the other type of content may merely be the stutterer telling the clinician what he thinks the clinician wants to hear.

It would also be possible to train the stutterer through biofeedback and operant methods to regulate his internal excitement levels (sustaining patterns that reflect both calm and emotionalism) during therapy to provide him with experiences of monitoring his newly acquired target behavior under varying internal emotional conditions. Our goals in such tactics would not be to teach the stutterer how to relax in the face of stimulating circumstances; but rather how to cope with such excitement, how to participate in and experience the emotional situations that are available in society, with the same relative fluency that the nonstutterer emits during states of emotional excitement. Excitement and emotions are not to be avoided, but are to be approached and dealt with as a fluent speaker would deal with them.

INSTATEMENT OF FLUENCY

Most people working in the operant area readily acknowledge that there are a number of ways to establish fluent speech in the clinic setting. Most of this early work focused on the overt motor speech behavior of the stutterer. The goal was speech that was free of stuttering.

RATE CONTROL

Starting with Flanagan, Goldiamond, and Azrin's (1958, 1959) early experimental work testing and demonstrating the operant nature of stuttering and the functions of several contingent stimuli (both aversive and positive), a series of therapies have emerged that are now known as Rate Control Therapy. Curlee and Perkins (1969), Perkins (1973a, 1973b), Ryan (1971), Ryan and Van Kirk (1973), Ryan and Van Kirk (1974) have been reporting fairly consistent success with the Flanagan et al. approach.

The Flanagan et al. studies provided a prototype in which delayed auditory feedback was used in a negative reinforcement paradigm. DAF is considered aversive. The stutterer is instructed that he may terminate this aversive DAF condition by slowing down his rate of speech, by prolonging and stretching the sounds, by sustaining his phonation so that there are no silent intervals between words, and by appropriate phrasing. The stutterer goes through a progression of delay intervals from 250 milliseconds to 0 milliseconds in 50 millisecond steps. As he progresses through shorter and shorter delays, his rate of talking increases until it approximates a normal conversational pattern. The Perkins programs and the Ryan programs employ different criteria of stutter-free speech for progressing through the delay intervals; but both arrive at a similar point in therapy for the stutterer. Eventually, the stutterer goes off the DAF-negative reinforcement program and faces the task of monitoring his fluency in real-life situations. In his Transfer and Maintenance programs, Ryan attempts to arrange for external positive reinforcement from family, friends, teachers, etc. Perkins arranges for the stutterer to periodically rate himself for fluency after he has spoken in specifically designated real-life situations.

Both Ryan and Perkins have also approached Rate Control Therapy without using the DAF recorder, but with only instructions and examples. By receiving approval for attempts to match the clinician's model, stutterers have learned to gradually shape a slowed-down rate of talking to conversational rates with results similar to those in the DAF program. However, both Ryan and Perkins report that the DAF program moves the stutterer along more rapidly.

Shames has used the DAF as a rate calibrator in a rate control program. In this tactic, the stutterer uses the DAF at a particular delay interval to help to establish a slow rate. He then goes off of the DAF until he can reach a number of criteria of stutter-free speech at that rate and delay interval. He returns to and leaves the DAF at progressively shorter intervals (and at associated faster rates), until he is talking in a normal conversational pattern, free of stuttering. Then the stutterer is at the same point in therapy as in the Perkins and Ryan programs—ready to monitor his fluency in real-life situations.

STRENGTHENING COEXISTING FLUENCY

Some therapy programs have been devised to increase the length of fluency responses that coexist with stuttering. Several different tactics have been explored. One approach has involved shaping longer fluent utterances, in terms of words, phrases, sentences, and free conversation. Another has tried to establish and strengthen fluency intervals in terms of amounts of time during which the stutterer speaks without stuttering.

Stuttering is not a target response for any type of consequation in such programs. Fluent speech is the only response that generates a contingent reaction from the clinician.

Rickard and Mundy (1965) shaped the fluency of a nine-year-old stutterer from short one- and two-word utterances to phrases, paragraphs, and free conversation. They gave points and approval for each class of response. When the goal of fluent speech with the clinician was reached, the stutterer's family was brought in to continue with the positive reinforcement activities. However, a follow-up study revealed that not all of the gains in fluency were maintained.

Leach (1969) employed a fluency interval program with a 12-year-old male stutterer. During 42 sessions, Leach paid the child two cents for every minute of talking time. After the first 15 minutes, he added an additional penny for each 15 seconds of fluency during the final 15 minutes of each session. Dysfluencies were eventually reduced to fewer than one per minute. However, follow-up studies again revealed that gains in fluency were not maintained after the experimental program was terminated.

Shaw and Shrum (1972) also reinforced fluency intervals with three children who stuttered. However, they permitted each child to select his own reinforcement (trading points for a preferred toy or candy). They used different fluency intervals for each child, based on the basal fluency interval rate of each. They also gave instructions to the children. One child was reinforced for every five seconds of fluency and two were reinforced for every ten seconds of fluency. Each child showed significant increases in his number of reinforcible fluency intervals and significant decrements in dysfluency. Only one child reached what was considered fluent speech.

In several short-term demonstration projects, Shames and several of his students have also explored the tactics of reinforcing fluency intervals. Kodish and Tucciarone (1973) developed a program for shaping progressively longer fluency intervals during a series of five 45-minute clinical interviews. From a basal fluency interval of 13 seconds, one adult stutterer reached a 38-second fluency interval during his fifth interview. The stutterer was given approval by the interviewer each time he reached his targeted fluency interval. When he reached that interval three consecutive times (i.e., 13 seconds of fluency, followed by 13 seconds of fluency, followed by another 13 seconds of fluency), the interval was increased in small time units. During the first two interviews, the fluency interval was increased in five-second steps. During the final three interviews, because the stutterer did not go beyond 29 seconds of fluency, the increase was reduced to one-second steps. The stutterer was then able to reach a 38-second fluency interval. Associated with these increases in fluency intervals was a decrease in dysfluencies. In the base rate interview, 179 dysfluencies by the stutterer were observed. This dropped to 32 dysfluencies in the final operant level session.

It is interesting to note that what could not be accomplished with a 5-second increase could be accomplished with a 1-second increase during the shaping of longer fluency intervals. The size of this time step in such a program may be a highly individual problem and it appears to be critical to a successful program. In another demonstration project an adult stutterer's fluency interval was lengthened by employing a response-cost paradigm (Witzel and Shulman, 1973).

During ten one-hour interviews, starting with a fluency interval of 30 seconds in Session 1, an adult stutterer was given one point for speaking fluently for that interval of time. If he stuttered during those 30 seconds he lost one point. When the stutterer could sustain his fluency interval for a continuous ten-minute period, the interval was increased in 15-second steps. The stutterer was also given an opportunity to gamble the next time for double the points each time he met a criterion. He could lose what he had accumulated for speaking fluently at a given time interval, or he could win double the points if he spoke fluently for that interval of time. It took five interviews for the stutterer to speak fluently for ten continuous minutes while being reinforced for every 30 seconds of fluency. In Session 8, the ten-minute criterion of fluency for a 45-second interval was reached. In Session 9, the 60-second fluency interval criterion was met.

During the ten interviews the stutterer could have gambled for double points 450 times. He did so about 70 percent of the time. He was successful in his gambles about 85 percent of the time. It was noted that the stutterer gambled more often later in the experiment, as the fluency time requirements became longer. This type of paradigm may be an analogue for the real-life gambles and expectations that a stutterer experiences, and emphasizes the importance of prior successful experiences with fluency in developing a commitment to future fluency.

Ryan (1971) and Ryan and Van Kirk (1973) have also reported on using programs that attempted to strengthen fluency. Their GILCU programs (Gradual Increase in Length and Complexity of Utterances) appeared to be as effective as their DAF programs in establishing fluency. They combine the reinforcement of a fluent utterance (one word, two words, etc.) with the reinforcement of a fluent time interval (30- and 45-second monologues). Marked decrements in stuttering have been observed to levels of less than 1 percent. At this point, their stutterers enter the maintenance and transfer phases of their therapy programs. These additional phases of therapy may account for Ryan and Van Kirk's higher success rates with this method for establishing fluency.

SUPPRESSION OF STUTTERING

Therapy programs designed to suppress stuttering are probably among the most controversial of all of the operant based activities. As such, they may appear to be minimally accommodating to traditional techniques. This is probably because the word "suppression" has been used almost interchangeably with the word "punishment." In the traditional operant framework, the punishment refers to a process that contains three designated elements—an *aversive* stimulus that has a *suppressive* effect on the response upon which it is *contingent*. Recently, workers have been willing to forsake the *aversive* element of that definition; they find they can comfortably work with a concept that includes only that the stimulus be *contingent* and that the effect be *suppressive*. Siegel has offered a highlighting hypothesis relative to this and states that any event that calls attention to the occurrence of a dysfluency will result in its reduction (1970).

Most of the research work carried out within a suppression paradigm has had broader implications than therapy. Results of these studies carry information about onset, prevention, and maintenance, as well as about therapy for stuttering. Only a few such studies were conceptualized exclusively as therapeutic tactics.

The original Flanagan et al. (1958) studies demonstrated that stuttering frequency could be reduced through contingent stimulation. The work started by Flanagan et al. was picked up and elaborated by

Martin and Siegel in a large-scale program of research on punishment and stuttering.

Siegel (1970) has summarized the results of these studies as follows:

> In the earliest experiments, electric shock was made the consequence of each stuttering; later verbal stimuli such as "wrong" were substituted. In more recent research the punishing stimulus has been a "time-out" period of several seconds in which the stutterer is not allowed to continue talking, or a "response-cost" method in which the stutterer loses points or money for each moment of stuttering. Most of the sessions have been conducted in the same experimental facility, with the subject alone in a room while the experimenter monitors from a control room. In some instances listeners have been added, and the subject has been asked to speak into a telephone. The specific response selected for modification has varied from a global "moment of stuttering" to a more particular behavior, such as a specific facial grimace or a vocal pattern. In general, and with due regard to differences among subjects, all of the techniques used—shock, verbal stimuli, time-out, response-cost—served as response depressants when arranged as a consequence of the response. This has been true with impressive consistency in both reading or speaking, whether the response was a particular behavior or simply "stuttering." . . . for the most part the results have not been permanent, and subjects quickly recovered their stuttering rates when the stimuli were withdrawn . . . or when they left the experimental facility. This is a familiar problem to speech pathologists. At present a major effort is being made to find ways to move the more fluent speech out of the laboratory and into more natural settings. (Pp. 681–682. Used by permission of the author.)

In addition to the studies on stutterers, Siegel and Martin undertook a series of projects that dealt with the dysfluencies of normal speakers. They explored the relative effectiveness of various types of contingent stimuli, verbal and nonverbal, on reading as well as on spontaneous speech. In general, they found that random aversive stimulation on both reading and speech had little suppressive effect. On the other hand, contingent aversive stimulation consistently resulted in reduced frequencies of dysfluency.

Suppressive effects were usually more pronounced for high frequency stutterers than for low frequency stutterers. Verbal reinforcers (words like "wrong") were more effective than electric shock. When the contingencies were withdrawn during speech, the frequency of dysfluencies did not return to its original rate. However, during reading, the original dysfluency rates were again approximated when the contingencies were withdrawn (Siegel and Martin, 1965a, 1965b; Siegel and Martin, 1966; Martin and Siegel 1966a, 1966b; Brookshire and Martin, 1967; Siegel and Martin, 1967; Quist and Martin, 1967; Martin, 1968; Siegel and Martin, 1968; Martin and Siegel, 1969) .

Three of the studies coming out of the University of Minnesota projects have implications for onset and prevention as well as for therapy. Brookshire (1969) and Brookshire and Eveslage (1969) explored the subject's history of punishment as a factor in its suppressive effects. The studies were done on normal adults and therefore extrapolation to the prevention of stuttering in children has to be a highly inferential process. Brookshire found that the suppressive effects of contingent aversive stimulation were reduced when it was preceded by random aversive stimulation of the same form. In the Brookshire and Eveslage study it was found that such antecedent random stimulation did not reduce the suppressive effects if it was of a different form than the contingent stimulation (i.e., noise during random stimulation; the word "wrong" during contingent stimulation).

These types of laboratory arrangements may well be an analogue of the real-life situation young developing stutterers encounter. When aversive control is prominent in a household, it is typically at the convenience of the parent, on an intermittent if not random schedule, and usually of the same form (i.e., shouting, spanking, loss of privilege, etc.). Such an analogue suggests reasons for the ineffectiveness and possibly detrimental effects of uncontrolled aversive stimulation in the home by parents. Such findings may also fit in with many of the traditionally held views of the dangers of punishment and its functions in the development of stuttering (Van Riper, 1937, Frick, 1951).

Halvorson (1971) also demonstrated the problems that can easily be encountered in contingent aversive stimulation. He first established the suppressive effects of punishment on the frequency of stuttering of three adult stutterers with a response-cost paradigm (the stutterer lost a point on a counter after each instance of stuttering). He then paired this procedure with positive reinforcement for the first fluent word following an instance of stuttering (the stutterer lost one point for stuttering and gained ten points for the first fluent word). The effect of pairing punishment with positive reinforcement was an increase in stuttering to its original rate. One way to get points is to stutter first and then say a fluent word. This experimental tactic may resemble the real-life situation of the developing stutterer. As Siegel (1970) points out, it is common to observe parents who first punish their child and then follow this with displays of affection. A child could easily learn that his emission of undesirable behavior is an effective way of generating affection and attention.

We could speculate that the parent and child may be conditioning one another in a most insidious way. Not only is the child learning, but so is the parent. The parent who "corrects" her stuttering child maintains her role of authority and wisdom; is the source of correction and information; can express her love and affection; can reaffirm her power to control her child's behavior; and keeps the child in a young, submissive, and dependent role. Such factors could be extremely powerful in maintaining the parent's behavior in such a circumstance.

Although all three of these studies (Brookshire, 1969; Brookshire and Eveslage, 1969; and Halvorson, 1971) are excellent laboratory studies of how contingent aversive stimulation may affect dysfluency and stuttering, they point up the differences between the laboratory and real life. Unless aversive stimulation can be employed in a controlled way, in terms of its scheduling, form, and relation with positive reinforcement, it can have detrimental effects. These studies may in fact contraindicate their use unless such careful control can be exercised.

Two suppression studies that were conceived only as explorations for their therapeutic value were carried out by Egolf et al. (1971) and by Blind et al. (1973). In the Egolf study, time-out procedures were employed as part of a stutterer's group therapy experience. Although the group of ten stutterers employed these T-O procedures for only five weeks, significant changes were observed. Each stutterer could talk as long as he was fluent (talking was viewed as positively reinforcing). If he stuttered, he had to relinquish the floor to the next group member. The average fluency time for the group increased from 20.8 seconds to 290.3 seconds. The average number of fluent words per stutterer increased from 33.4 to 583.6 words. In some instances, the fluency intervals were 30 times longer during T-O segments than during noncontingent segments.

In another therapy study, the contingent suppressive consequence consisted of having the clinician reiterate the word stuttered by the stutterer (Blind et al., 1973). Results of this tactic with 17 adult stutterers showed significant decrements in stuttering. Pre-therapy frequencies ranged from 4.9 percent to 50.1 percent or a mean of 15.8 percent. Sixteen of the stutterers reduced their stuttering to less than 1 percent (as described in greater detail in Chapter Seven under Form Program Three).

SELF-RESPONSIBILITY

Most of us would agree that therapy is not a passive process. Events do not occur all by themselves. Things happen because people help them to happen. However, stutterers often approach this rather awesome experience and their somewhat authoritative clinicians in a posture of waiting to be ministered to. They come saying, "Help me," "Do things to me to make me speak better." Too frequently, we fall in with such seductive pleas because it elevates us to omnipotence. However, clinicians have been observed in a "do it for yourself" posture, in an almost rejecting attitude of the stutterer's need to be helped toward that final goal of independence and self-responsibility. An ultimate goal of therapy is to have the stutterer become independent of the clinician and the clinic, to be able to act for himself and to cope with his system of living. Ultimate goals, however, are not reached in the first session. Most stutterers will have to be nurtured during therapy toward that end and not abruptly shocked into it during a diagnostic. Therefore, self-responsibility as a class of responses warrants considerable discussion. This type of response may well be the key to the long-range success of therapy.

As with other classes of responses that are considered within the framework of operant conditioning, self-responsibility must be operationally defined and behaviorally described as precisely as possible. Behavioral responses that reflect self-responsibility must be designated, opportunities for their occurrence must be arranged, and consequences for their emission must be provided. The first step in such a conceptualization is to say what we mean by self-responsibility. In the context of therapy for stuttering, we mean that the stutterer eventually will do for himself what had previously been done for him by others (clinician, parents, spouse, peers, etc.), who become a part of his therapy regime and play a role in strengthening desirable responses and in weakening undesirable responses. The stutterer is taught to provide the occasions for his target behavior and to consequate his own behavior. The when and how of learning self-responsibility behavior may not be a simple matter of instruction, prodding, or brief discussion. It may in and of itself require a conditioning procedure that is separate from responses more topographically related to stuttering. It is a part of the therapy problem. Therefore, it does not represent a detour, but rather the acquisition of a pertinent class of responses that makes the therapy more cohesive and durable.

Self-responsibility behavior does not occur in a vacuum of responses. It is a class of responses about another class of responses. The stutterer learns to be responsible for dealing with (by occasioning and by consequating) other aspects of his behavior that are more topographically related to stuttering. Eventually, the stutterer will be faced with monitoring his fluency, arranging for real-life talking situations, and evaluating his behavior on his own.

The tactics for reaching this goal can be affected by a number of variables. A technology about self-monitoring and self-reinforcement has been developing in therapeutic contexts outside the field of stuttering therapy. This field of research has focused primarily on tactics of self-reinforcement, but it has also considered certain characteristics of the subjects. The problems that have been studied include weight reduction (Quick, 1973; Bellack et al., 1973; Mahoney et al., 1973); smoking (McFall, 1970; Rozensky, 1973); homosexual behavior (Rehm and Rozensky, 1973); scratching behavior (Watson et al., 1972); disruptive classroom behavior (Bolsted and Johnson, 1972); stealing (Epstein and Peterson, 1973); insomnia (Bootzin, 1972); self-mutilation (Ernst, 1973); alcohol consumption (Sobell and Sobell, 1973); and self-concept (Rehm and Marston, 1968). By systematically varying conditions of self-control and external control, it has been possible to determine the relative reliance on external contingencies for changing behavior in desirable ways. As in the work with stutterers, the ultimate goal is to develop tactics that enable a person to manage his problems on his own. Kanfer and Phillips (1966) refer to this process as Instigation Therapy. In such an approach, the clinician helps the client to plan his therapy and then supervises him as he carries it out in his own environment. The early work in this area demonstrated the parallels between external reinforcement and self-reinforcement via similar scheduling effects (Kanfer and Marston, 1963; Marston, 1964, 1965; Kanfer, 1967). Kanfer (1970a; 1079b) and Kanfer and Karoly (1972) offered a three-stage theoretical model for self-reinforcement. First is the monitoring and attending stage, which tells the client that he behaved (or will behave) in a certain way. Second, the client evaluates his behavior against some criterion. Third, the client consequates his behavior. To apply this model to therapy for stuttering, the stutterer: (1) attends to his speech (i.e., a predesignated type of response, such as an instant of stuttering, or an interval of fluency, or a modification of the form of stuttering); (2) evaluates his behavior against some predesignated criterion (i.e., a particular fluency interval, or a specific way of modifying stuttering); and (3) approves or disapproves or uses some tangible form of consequence, depending on whether he met his criterion. The application of this model to stuttering therapy is quite apparent. For effective carryover of clinical fluency, stutterers may have to learn systematically these three phases of self-regulation. Perhaps we should actively acknowledge this as a typical phase of our therapy.

Coming out of this research area have been some fairly consistent results and strong suggestions for tactics. It appears that it is more effective to monitor desirable behavior than to monitor undesirable behavior (Mahoney et al., 1973). Related to this finding is that it is more effective to positively reinforce than to punish. This conclusion has a direct bearing on our work with stutterers. It would appear to tell us that it would be more effective to positively self-reinforce fluency than to punish oneself for stuttering. Obviously, monitoring stuttering is going to lead to self-punishment and monitoring fluency should lead to positive reinforcement. However, the process of monitoring (attending, counting, and getting feedback about the emission of behavior) may be independent of the process of evaluation and may not necessarily automatically trigger an evaluation. Also, even if a stutterer learns to monitor, and learns to evaluate, as two independent processes and types of behavior responses, he may still need to learn to consequate formally his behavior, either verbally or in some more tangible way. Training in each of these three stages and processes during therapy is quite feasible. Perkins (1973a and b) has taught stutterers to manage their own DAF programs. Ryan (1970) teaches stutterers to count instances of stuttering for certain of his programs, thereby giving them feedback about their behavior. Such training in self-monitoring, evaluating, and consequating may at first be approached by having the stutterers publicly monitor, evaluate, and consequate. For example, the stutterer says: (1) "I stuttered"; (2) "I didn't want to stutter"; (3) "I lose a point on the counter"; or (1) "I was fluent for five minutes"; (2) "I met my criterion"; (3) "That's good, now I can go on to the next step." When the clinician is satisfied that the stutterer can emit these behaviors, they can be dealt with as covert thoughts and judged for their occurrence by the emission of other related behaviors (i.e., "going on to the next step," in the example above). As simplistic as the above illustrations may appear to be, they may be effective events in maintaining newly acquired target behavior. There has been some additional evidence that monitoring "the intent to respond" even before the response is emitted is more effective than monitoring after a response has been made (Bellack et al., 1973).

Another tactic that could affect self-reinforcement programs is the scheduling of feedback about overall progress toward a goal. Some researchers have concluded that the immediate effects of individual instances of a contingency are all that is necessary (Quick, 1973), while others feel that such overall feedback, if clear, understandable, and goal-oriented, can provide additional support for self-regulated therapy (Locke et al., 1968).

It has also been found that the more motivated clients do better in self-regulation (Kolb et al., 1968; McFall, 1970; McFall and Hammen, 1971). However, the measurement of motivation can be a major problem and often is judged by a few answers to a questionnaire, or subjectively from imprecise interview material. The motivations of the stutterer to change his speech have been commented on clinically and indirectly, but have not been the subject for formal research.

Many years ago, Abbott (1947) suggested that stutterers had strong unconscious motivations to keep their symptoms because of guilt over their repressed hostility toward listeners. Motivation was viewed as an internal state of the stutterer.

In a behavioral framework, motivation is viewed as a function of external operations and is thusly described. Usually deprivation procedures, as in social deprivation, water deprivation, etc., are described as procedures employed by an external agent to increase the effectiveness of a particular reinforcer (i.e., water or socialization). Such procedures are interpreted as motivational operations. Shames and Sherrick (1963) and later Rubin and Culatta (1971) comment on the "positive payoffs" and the "excuse for failure" as possible external motivating operations that help to maintain stuttering.

Although motivation does not guarantee success, the lack of it almost insures failure. An important clinical question for us is whether we can help a stutterer change if he is not strongly motivated. Can we help an unmotivated stutterer develop a real desire to change the way he talks socially so that the results of reinforcement tactics can be carried over into the stutterer's nonclinical world?

One study of carryover (Blind et al., 1972) has some direct implications for programming and operationalizing tactics that are directed toward motivating the stutterer. Blind et al. found that those stutterers who sustained their clinical fluency after terminating their formal clinical program were those who experienced profound changes in life styles. Births, marriages, deaths, divorces, and changes in occupation were more frequently observed in this group. Many of these events were not under the stutterers' control. However, they were able to cope with these changes as fluent speakers. This finding suggests that we should provide time during therapy for discussing the stutterer's life system and arrange for experiences that will help the stutterer become aware of the meaningfulness and significance of becoming a fluent speaker. It is possible that special thematic content programs can be devised that are directed toward such material, or that nonprogrammed discussions can be held early in therapy or as the stutterer is establishing his new speech responses. Such tactics could serve to motivate the stutterer and perhaps enhance the immediate reinforcement tactics of the clinician for responses that may lead to more general life goals. The development of self-responsibility and carryover procedures could well depend on these larger motivational operations and issues.

Still another variable that may be important is the client's perception of how much control he exerts over what happens to him. Rotter (1966) has developed a measure of Internal-External Locus of Control, and it has been suggested that clients who consider themselves in control of their destinies (and who score high on the Internal Scale) do better when external controls are removed.

There is a strong suggestion in this literature that locus of control may be a personality variable. Some people will always need a measure of external contingent support for sustaining target behavior. Others may find external control quite aversive and, in a therapeutic context, they may thrive on self-regulation and become casualties if placed in an external control regimen.

Bellack and Tillman (1973) have devised a simple memory-recognition behavioral test that identifies the self-reinforcement tendencies of people. In this test, subjects are asked to evaluate the accuracy of their performance, or the confidence they have that they have been correct. Rozensky (1974) explored the predictive value of this test in a therapeutic weight reduction program. He found that "high self-reinforcers" lost more weight in a self-control program than "low self-reinforcers." He also found that "low self-reinforcers" lost more weight in an externally controlled program.

This is an area that still needs a great deal of research, and as yet has not been related to the problems of the stutterer (Bandura, 1967; Mahoney, 1972a; Lefcourt, 1966; Kiesler, 1966).

As our tactics for instating and establishing desirable behavior in the stutterer may be becoming less of a clinical problem, *the need to sustain that behavior* over a long period of time may start to capture our attention in a more systematic way (Goldiamond, 1965). As self-responsibility and self-reinforcement become a more refined clinical process as part of a larger system of therapy, then the various tactics just discussed will have to be applied to the problem of therapy for stuttering. The stutterer's motivation, his history of self-reinforcement, his sense of internal control, and the methods used for establishing fluency may all influence decisions regarding the timing, scheduling, and forms of external as well as self-regulated activities in his therapy.

GROUP THERAPY

More often than not group therapy for stuttering has been used to relieve shortages of time and personnel, rather than for its merits and qualitative aspects. Until recently very little has been written describing the group situation as a therapeutic process for stuttering. And yet, in public schools as well as hospitals and clinics, group therapy may be as frequently encountered as individual therapy. Most of us grope blindly for a way of characterizing and implementing the relation between concurrent group and individual therapy. In some programs, stutterers might initiate their therapy in a group situation in which they share past experiences, desensitize one another, and plan and implement strategies for controlling their stuttering. They may form teams for engaging in activities outside of the group and then report back on their progress and problems. The group becomes the central organizing core around which all therapy is planned, discussed, implemented, and evaluated. On occasion, if a member develops a special problem, he may be invited to concurrently participate in individual therapy. Such individual sessions may deal with the management of stuttering behavior that has not responded to the group process or with deeper emotional problems that the group process may have brought to the stutterer's awareness. Individual sessions then take on the character of psychotherapy and counseling. However, even with the concurrent approach of individual and group therapy, the group session leads individual therapy.

Group therapy has also been used as a supplement or as a carryover phase of individual therapy. Typically in such orientations, it is during the individual session that the stutterer plans, discusses, implements, and evaluates his progress. The group session is employed, mainly, if at all, as the place to try out new skills, to habituate a new target response, and to discuss with other stutterers ideas that may have had their birth in the individual session. The group is a proving ground and a way station to carryover outside the clinic. Group therapy in this orientation follows rather than leads individual therapy. In some instances, group and individual therapy are phased, with individual therapy used to establish a new speech response, and group therapy used for carryover. The functions of each type of session may remain fixed throughout therapy.

Very little has been systematically done with group therapy in the operant area. By systematic is meant the identification of certain group processes in the forms of group-evoking stimuli; occasions for talking that are a function of group interaction; reinforcing events that emanate from the group; and target responses relative to the group process and group membership that are somehow unique or more easily arranged in a group situation. We are thinking here that group therapy should not be a series of individual therapy encounters involving a clinician-stutterer dyad, while the other stutterers in the group sit and wait their turn. We are thinking here of such interactive behaviors as sharing, attending, listening, caring, leading, following, cooperating, being supportive, evaluative, or critical; or such procedures as counting and monitoring, and evaluating and reinforcing one another's behavior. These behaviors could be extremely therapeutic for the group members and can be arranged only in the group situation.

"The Shaping Group" has been the most programmatic approach to developing group conditioning tactics as a process of therapy for stuttering. Leith and Uhlemann (1970a; 1970b; 1970c; 1972) in a series of projects have focused on both stuttering and interpersonal behaviors among stutterers in a group situation within a conditioning framework. Their purpose is to modify specific behaviors that interfere with a group member's interpersonal relations. Stutterers set their own behavioral goals with help from one another; instructed in the principles of operant conditioning, they are trained in providing consequences for each other's behavior. Members become familiar with one another's goals and become agents of reinforcement for one other. They give feedback to each other about the impact of behavior. Leith and Uhlemann (1970a; 1970b) report on their results with nine stutterers. These stutterers showed changes over time in terms of within-group processes. However, changes in stuttering and in self-concept were variable among the subjects. It was felt that lengthy intersession intervals may have been a factor in the limited effectiveness of their program. The importance of these projects is not necessarily in the results, but rather in the description of the procedures. At best, group situations are a complicated, dynamic, and difficult system to describe and operationalize. Leith and Uhlemann have demonstrated the possibilities of structuring in a very complicated system of interpersonal interactions. The fact that they experienced only limited success in changing the stutterer's behavior means that further systematic experimentation is in order. But they have evolved the system for that program of research within the particular independent and dependent variables they have focused on. Eventually this research may result in group tactics that may be clinically effective.

In another type of group therapy project, a time-out from reinforcement paradigm was employed with ten adult male stutterers by Egolf et al. (1971). Although this study was presented earlier as an example of a suppression study, it also has implications for group therapeutic tactics. The stutterers were highly verbal, and talking in the group appeared to be a positive experience. Each stutterer was told that he could talk as long as he was fluent. If he stuttered he had to relinquish the floor to another member of the group. Each member had an opportunity to talk during a session. Part of each group session involved a time-out contingency. Although the group met only once a week, the effects of the time-out procedure were profound. During the noncontingency segment, the mean fluency time was 20.8 seconds for the group. This increased to a mean fluency time of 290.3 seconds during the time-out segments, for an increase of more than ten times the noncontingent fluency. Word output during time-out increased almost 20 times over word output during noncontingent segments. It changed from a mean of 33.4 words per stutterer to a mean of 583.6 words per stutterer. It was concluded that high frequency stutterers did not do so well as low frequency stutterers. It was also felt that a shaping procedure could be employed by having each stutterer establish his own fluency interval base rate, in order to gradually increase the length of each stutterer's fluency interval. In this type of project, the occasion for the stutterer's responses was the group audience situation. The target response was an instance of stuttering. The source and form of reinforcement was the approval from the other group members; and the contingency was a time-out from that source of group social reinforcement.

Another elaborate program of research on group therapy for stuttering is the Token Economy approach of Andrews and Ingham. (Anddrews, 1971; Andrews and Ingham, 1971; Ingham and Andrews, 1971; Ingham and Winkler, 1972). Their conceptualization of the group was much broader in scope and application than the usual group therapy session format. They attempted to evolve a microsociety of stutterers within a hospital setting. In this society, stutterers had to earn tokens to purchase some of the necessities and luxuries available for a three-week stay in the hospital (i.e., cigarettes, desserts, and soft beds). Each stutterer's base rate for syllable output and fluent speech was progressively changed toward normal stutter-free speech. At specified times and occasions during the day the stutterer could earn tokens for doing 10 percent better than his base rate at that time. Of 39 stutterers who went through this program, all showed marked reductions in stuttering. A series of follow-up studies suggested that the use of DAF was the most effective of several procedures employed for establishing fluent speech. Also it was felt that follow-up therapy experiences would enhance the changes in behavior achieved during hospitalization. This particular approach to therapy is intriguing from the methodological standpoint of trying to achieve significant control of the stutterer's behavior on an around-the-clock basis. But from another standpoint, the societal concept as the context for therapy may get us closer to the contingencies of secondary social and monetary reinforcers that operate in real life. As in the Leith and Uhlemann projects, this program of research has evolved the format of contingencies, responses, and consequences necessary for further experimentation. In the future, these projects may have to give closer attention to the occasions and the evoking stimuli for the responses being consequated in the token economy setting.

PROGRAMMING THE OCCASIONS
FOR CARRYOVER

Thus far in this chapter we have considered the possible ways that the principles of operant conditioning could accommodate traditional theories about stuttering. We have also discussed some of the various tactics that could be generated to establish fluency, to modify feelings and beliefs, and to establish self-responsibility. All these issues point in the direction of, or have implications for, the clinical process known as "carryover." This is a process of transferring the behavior the stutterer has acquired in the clinic situation to the everyday routine of nonclinical life. We have talked about establishing responses and monitoring responses; now we must examine the stimulus circumstances during which these responses occur. The first element in the operant paradigm is the occasion for the emission of target behavior.

Typically, the primary occasion for target responses has been the presence of the clinician in a small clinical cubicle. Getting the target response out of that fairly protected and socially remote situation may involve a lot of planning and social engineering.

Ryan (1970) in the transfer and maintenance phase of his therapy has tried systematically to arrange to transfer the stutterer's fluency behavior. He programs the occasions for responses by gradually changing the stimulus components of the occasion. For example, he gradually increases the size of the audience, he gradually takes the stutterer out of the room and into corridors and other rooms, he introduces the telephone, he programs the family to provide the consequences he formerly provided, and he introduces unfamiliar people as an audience. The principle is to transfer stimulus control over fluency.

Perkins (1973a and b) has also attempted to organize the occasions for monitoring fluency outside of the clinic. In his program, the stutterer moves through a progressively more difficult series of talking situations and rates himself later about various aspects of his performance. Rating is an attempt to inject a periodic and viable consequence for monitoring a fluent pattern of speech into the stutterer's real life.

The occasions to be considered in monitoring fluency during carryover would logically be related to those occasions for stuttering that were sampled during the initial evaluations of the problem. For example, if in the initial evaluation we observed that a stutterer had difficulty talking on the telephone, then we most assuredly would want to provide some experiences for monitoring the stutterer's fluency on the telephone.

For the most part the selection of these occasions for monitoring target behavior as a formal part of therapy have been arbitrary. They should derive from the individual problems of each stutterer. If our observations of the stutterer's self-monitoring of fluency behavior have been extensive we should be able to arrange a series of experiences, probably from least to most difficult.

The specific occasions that have received the most attention and are viable for systematic carryover tactics are listed in Chapter Three, Table 3.1. Logically, occasions significant in the evaluation of the problem should be considered for their functions in carryover.

For carryover, the tactics in general would be to arrange a progression of experiences, within each category of circumstance, beginning with those associated with the lowest frequency of stuttering and progressing to those associated with the highest frequency of stuttering (on the assumption that it is easier to monitor fluency under conditions of least stuttering and more difficult to monitor fluency under conditions of most stuttering) . Such an arrangement is suggestive of a hierarchy of stimulus conditions not based on anxiety, but rather on observations of stuttering behavior or ability to monitor new target behavior.

Each of the circumstances listed in Table 3.1 can be approached through discussions, role playing, acting out, or realistically encountered outside the clinic, to provide the stutterer with experiences with his target behavior under varying degrees and types of stimulus occasions.

Which occasions should be systematically introduced into the therapy program depends on the stutterer and the relations that have been observed between the circumstances and the stutterer's ability to emit and to monitor his target behavior. It is quite conceivable that for some stutterers only one or two of these occasions may be factors in carryover. Judgments and therapeutic programming should be made to fit the individual's case. However, standardized methods for probing the significance of these variables for each stutterer would appear to be a necessary clinical endeavor and perhaps is of greater functional importance than the time-honored case history and adaptation tests that are so frequently done during diagnostic evaluations.

EFFECTS OF SCHEDULING
ON CARRYOVER

One of the most important kinds of information coming out of the laboratory experiments on conditioning of animals and humans deals with the effects of various schedules of contingent stimulation on behavioral acquisition and its extinction.

There are basically two schedules of reinforcement. One is continuous reinforcement, in which a consequence is provided after each occurrence of a target response. The second is an intermittent schedule, in which consequences are provided on some noncontinuous schedule. On this schedule, every target response is not consequated. Intermittent schedules can be based on the passage of a time interval, so that the consequence is provided after the first target response is emitted following a fixed or variable amount of time. Consequences can also be intermittently provided after a fixed or variable number of target responses have been emitted. This is known as a Ratio Schedule.

The scheduling of external reinforcement, and its withdrawal and replacement by self-reinforcement procedures, may have direct implications for the process of clinical carryover. Tactics involving a sequence of experiences that progress from external support, to self-support, to a point of no explicit support for newly acquired target behavior could generate a clinical technology of its own. Listeners do not usually reinforce fluency behavior per se in their conversational partners. Responses that were explicitly consequated in the clinic setting routine are non-discriminated in natural social settings. If anything, such responses get attached to other aspects of the person's nonclinical behavior, such as the content of what he is talking about or his style of interacting. Whether this is a process of extinction, of transferring stimulus control, or of reinforcing a larger class of responses of which fluency is only one element, is not clearly understood. The relations among such processes in a clinical context are also open to speculation and hypothesizing.

Although responses that are acquired through continuous reinforcement have the fastest acquisition rate, they also have the most rapid extinction rate when reinforcement is withdrawn. Such rapid acquisition may have very desirable effects on a stutterer's motivation and commitment to therapy early in treatment. In a shaping procedure, this seems to be the most effective schedule for successively approximating some final form of behavior. However, once that behavior is established, its durability may require that a shift to an intermittent schedule be arranged. Thus far, there has been no research on schedule effects or schedule tactics as they relate to clinical carryover. It may well be that a progression from continuous reinforcement to fixed intermittent reinforcement to variable intermittent reinforcement would have optimal clinical effects for sustaining fluency. It may also be that a combination of ratio and interval schedules is appropriate, as in the Ryan and Van Kirk therapy programs. The need for such clinical research is clearly present and may be a factor in the current success rates being reported.

SUMMARY

Although at times the operant model has been placed in opposition to various theoretical positions, we have attempted to show that such polarity in placement is not valid. The operant model can exist in a complementary relationship with many existing theories of human behavior. Such complementarity is especially useful in planning therapeutic programs. Theories suggest which behaviors are appropriate target responses for change and the operant model provides the blueprint for operationally bringing about the change. Because of this we have labeled the operant model as an accommodating model. It can accommodate many existing theories and ideas related to stuttering and human behavior.

Reviewed in this chapter were a large number of studies in behavior modification including studies designed to investigate the modification of stuttering. The sheer number of studies provides testimony in support of the heuristic value of the operant model. For this reason we have labeled the operant model as generative. It has been responsible for generating a plethora of studies. Heuristic value alone may serve to establish the value of the operant model. We believe, however, that the model has surpassed this single criterion. Results from the studies reviewed show that, in general, behavior was modified in the direction sought by researchers and subjects or by clinicians and clients. While we have no conclusive evidence to say that the operant approach is definitely superior to other approaches, we can say that operant researchers have publicly and in detail made available their procedures and results against which future comparisons of efficacy can be made.

11

··

Concluding
Comments

At the beginning of this book, it was suggested that all extant therapies for stuttering should be scrutinized with a common set of criteria to determine the individual merits of each. Several questions were posed for this purpose. It was further suggested that hard data should form the core of such assessments rather than the clinical experiences, anecdotes, and criticisms of a few experts. A particular therapy should stand on its own merits and data, and not survive because of the weaknesses perceived in opposing or parallel points of view. The six questions we will now apply to the operant therapies were designed to embrace the major issues that have to be faced in selecting a particular therapy. Hopefully, they are equally applicable to any therapy for stuttering and no therapy that may be examined thusly will suffer because of any inadequacies in the questions. Although some of our comments may be redundant, they are worth bringing together for a concluding discussion, to point up where we are and where we may be going.

*RELATIONS
TO THEORETICAL
POINTS OF VIEW*

The principles of operant conditioning are atheoretical. This may be considered a weakness because it implies an incompleteness in the approach. As a set of therapy principles, operant conditioning lacks content and does not describe the nature of the problem for which therapy is to be provided. Operant conditioning depends on other theoretically based orientations for its content. It tells us how to change stuttering behavior, and it guides us to antecedent and consequent events that may control the occurrence of stuttering, but it does not necessarily tell us what to change. Our only guideline to content from the operant framework is the temporal equation of the law of effect.

But this atheoretical nature of operant conditioning may also be perceived as a strength, since it can be legitimately applied to the observable events associated with a number of theoretical views of stuttering and of therapy. As a meta-method, it can accommodate and be applied to traditional content theories and therapies for stuttering. When this has been done, it has resulted in greater systematizing and description of that traditional approach. Much of the mystery and artistry of therapy can be better understood and implemented when its processes are operationally defined, in terms of the contingencies that influence the behaviors of both the stutterer and the clinician.

*DOES THIS POINT OF VIEW
LEAD TO STRATEGIES OF THERAPY
AND PROVIDE A DESCRIPTION
OF OPERATIONAL TACTICS?*

Probably the most significant strength of operant-based therapies is their openness and descriptiveness. The various ways these principles have been applied to therapy have been described in detail, are easily understood because of their descriptiveness; and exist primarily in a context of operational tactics. It is an empirical, tactical, response-contingent, data-oriented context of activity that is most appropriate and suitable for understanding and implementing much of what goes on during therapy. It is not an arm-chair, theorizing approach to therapy that speculates about dynamics and processes. It does not involve a great deal of inference and theoretical interpretation. The basic requirement is that the clinician formulate and implement a hypothesis about some aspect of the stutterer's behavior and how he might provide consequences for that behavior to change it in some desirable fashion. The clinician formulates and tests therapeutic tactical hypotheses. The observed changes in the stutterer's behavior will promptly tell him of the validity of the hypothesis and whether he is on the right tactical track, or whether he needs to revise what he is doing.

IS THERE A CHANGE
IN STUTTERING AND IN BEHAVIOR
ASSOCIATED WITH IT?

The operant approach has sometimes been criticized because it has been too narrow in scope. The primary focus has been on stuttering behavior, with the result that several methods for reducing stuttering have emerged. The rate control therapies, the suppression and highlighting methods, and the fluency interval therapies have each been effective in reducing stuttering, sometimes rather quickly. The general impact of the results of this focus on stuttering behavior is the realization that there may be a number of ways to reduce stuttering, that it does not necessarily have to take a long time to accomplish, and that the most serious issues in therapy lie in developing strategies of carryover rather than strategies for changing speech behavior.

Behaviors that are related to or affect stuttering have received far less attention than the stuttering response itself. Our own work on consequating the content themes emitted by adult stutterers during interviews and modifying parent-child verbal interactions could be considered steps in the direction of these related behaviors. These two particular approaches to therapy were conceptualized as tactics for reducing stuttering. But these thematic and interactive responses may actually be manipulated as behaviors independent of stuttering, and be more functional if conceptualized as separate but related target behavior, or as an issue in carryover. Although parent-child interactions and adult content themes may be important aspects of the problem of stuttering, they may not always be the appropriate behavior to be targeted for manipulation as a way of reducing stuttering. Poor parent-child verbal interactions may constitute significant occasions for sustaining fluency that has been established in a more direct fashion (i.e., rate control, suppression, fluency reinforcement). Consideration of what the stutterer's beliefs are and what he says about himself and his speech may be different in content and may be of greater significance after fluency has been established than during the process of changing the motor aspects of his speech. A stutterer may talk about himself and his problems differently as a fluent speaker than he would as a stuttering speaker.

The biofeedback research of Treon et al. (1972) and the work on GSR by Reed and Lingwall (1973) and by Gray and England (1968) might also be significant beginnings for clinical biofeedback tactics that focus on emotional behavior related to stuttering.

In general, the emotional aspects of stuttering and of stutterers who develop fluent patterns of talking are not well understood and need a considerable amount of thought, hypothesizing, and empirical data. Once these relations are understood, we can face the issue of developing tactics for applying this information to therapy. Still another type of behavior that is related to therapy for the problem of stuttering is that of the stutterer's independence and self-responsibility. If the stutterer's new speech responses, beliefs, and perceptions of himself are to be sustained, they must be sustained without the support of the clinician. Deliberate and systematic training in self-monitoring, self-evaluation, and self-reinforcement may be the way to establish the stutterer's independence and freedom from the need for external, clinical support.

There may be a prototypical model of significant issues in therapy emerging from this discussion. Although the order of the list below does not suggest a strict sequence, each item may be important to successful therapy:

1. Instate fluent speech.
2. Establish a belief system and self-perception in a speaker that are congruent with fluent speaking behavior.
3. Train the stutterer in self-monitoring, self-evaluation and self-reinforcement so that he may regulate his therapy on his own.
4. Program the occasions for carryover to insure significant experiences outside the clinic with his newly acquired target behaviors.

These four processes can be arranged in a number of ways. They may take a number of forms, vary in sequence, and involve different conditioning programs for different stutterers. But it may be that there is a universal, although variable, structure of these four processes that underlies effective therapy. The validity of this hypothesis is yet to be systematically tested in the context of clinical research.

CAN THE THERAPY BE EVALUATED?

Because of the laboratory history of operant conditioning the importance and dependence on empirical data is built into the system. Changes in frequency of target responses are the primary data for assessing the efficacy of a particular therapeutic tactic. The evaluative data are there, are available, and are explicit. They need only be tabulated and interpreted. However, there may be a number of important events going on during therapy that are not accounted for by frequency tabulations. Processes of interaction, awareness and cognition, countercontrol and resistance, styles, sequence analysis of content themes, emotional excitement levels, first insight and low frequency behaviors (i.e., severe but infrequent stuttering) may be significant aspects of therapy and may operate outside of the usual frequency of occurrence system for evaluating therapy. The significance of these events during therapy has not been determined and it appears that tabulating the frequency of their occurrence may not provide the answers. We still have to determine what can be predicted from such events relative to process and outcome of therapy. In general, insofar as stuttering behavior is concerned (as separated from the larger issue of the total stuttering problem), this can be evaluated for desirable change and assessed for efficacy of tactics with frequency of occurrence data. However, even these assessments must go beyond the behavior that is observed in the therapy room. It should include long-term follow-up data in the social milieu and real-life encounters of each stutterer.

CAN THE THERAPY BE REVISED IN A SYSTEMATIC AND ORDERLY FASHION?

Earlier in the book, it was urged that we not become trial-and-error technique hunters, but rather that we learn the principles of operant conditioning that can be translated into a number of clinical tactics. The principles and tactics involved here are those of arranging and providing occasions and consequences for specific responses emitted by the stutterer. Although there are a finite number of types of paradigms for occasions and consequences that a clinician can provide or arrange, there are an infinite number of forms that the paradigms can take. These paradigms are designed to either strengthen desirable behavior or weaken undesirable behavior. Judgments about revision of tactics therefore are directed in an orderly fashion to one of several issues within the operant paradigm. Revisions can involve retaining the same type of consequence (i.e., to increase a behavior), but revising its form; for example, using money instead of approval. Revisions can involve changing the type of consequence and, as a result, the target behavior; for example, changing from approval for 15 seconds of fluency to a format of disapproval for each instance of stuttering. Revision can involve changing the occasion for a target response; for example, instead of asking questions to evoke target responses, instructing the stutterer to tell a brief story to evoke verbal responses. Revisions can involve changing the schedule for providing consequences; for example, switching from a continuous schedule to an intermittent schedule. The strategies for revisions are not trial and error; they are developed within a system that has rules and procedures for assessing the effectiveness of a particular paradigm, for studying the response frequencies and rates of the stutterer, and for systematically varying the arrangement until a satisfactory result is obtained or until all viable strategies have been exhausted.

DOES THE THERAPY ACCOUNT FOR THE SOCIAL AND EMOTIONAL CONTEXT OF THE PROBLEM?

This is basically a question of whether the changes in stuttering that are observed in the clinic setting carry over into the stutterer's life system away from the therapist. Strategies for carryover and the assessment of outcome of therapy must be considered from both a methodological and a substantive standpoint. Methodologically (Perkins, 1973a and b; Ryan, 1973) almost no therapy until recently contained within its structure any strategy for achieving carryover of fluency. Possibly this was due to the pessimism among professionals about the possibility of ever having the stutterer become fluent, even in therapy. In short, the emergence of fluency seemed so remote that carryover was always beyond the range of visibility and thus ignored. As clinicians have become more successful in evoking fluency in stutterers the carryover problem has emerged. There are also the practical problems involved in incorporating carryover in a therapy program. It is expensive and time-consuming for former stutterers to return to clinics when indeed they see no need for it. It is also difficult to monitor their behavior outside the clinic. Usually it involves the participation of others, either directly, or indirectly, when the stutterer covertly records his conversations with them. Adding willing or unwilling participants complicates the implementation and monitoring procedures. Thus even a good design for carryover may flounder because the clinician cannot easily control situations outside of the clinic.

At another level carryover goals are often minimized because of the nature of stuttering. People simply do not die from stuttering. With other disorders, particularly physical diseases where a reoccurrence might be fatal, both professionals and patients are extremely vigilant about the disorder after successful treatment.

Notwithstanding the problems involved with carryover, we believe that plans for its implementation should be included in any therapy program to the extent that both clinician and client are aware that it is a part of treatment; specifically, the most important part. Thus, a client who is unwilling to agree to participate in certain activities outside the clinic, or who fails to agree to return periodically to the clinic after treatment, is essentially not a serious candidate for therapy. Commitment by both the clinician and the stutterer to carryover strategies and to follow-up evaluations is essential to understanding the nature of the therapeutic experience and to preventing possible relapses.

FINAL REMARKS

Beyond our attempts to relate the operant approach to some questions about its general effectiveness, we have become aware of the impact it has had on processes of therapy, both operant and nonoperant. Insofar as nonoperant therapies are concerned, there has been a significant systematizing effect. Traditionalists are beginning to ask questions about their procedures. They are seeing the need to document and to describe. They have become less casual about establishing specific goals, more specific and precise in measuring events, more descriptive in analyzing interactional systems, more discriminating in determining pertinent and relevant events. Many nonoperant therapists are wondering if some of the "do's" and "don'ts" of therapy are purely myths. They are aware of the need to document clinical observation and have become sharper and more skillful observers of the problem. Hopefully, they have become more comfortable in focusing on observable behavior and less guilty about their difficulties in dealing with the less observable feelings of the stutterer. Each of these effects, perhaps coincidentally, is an integral aspect of operant tactics and principles. But they appear to be suitable for any therapeutic approach to stuttering.

In addition to these impacts on nonoperant therapy, the operant approach has some obvious implications for operant-based therapy as well. One of these is the goal of therapy. The goal is not merely stuttering that is reduced in frequency or severity, or changed in form, but speech that is free of stuttering. It is further felt that the stutterer's perceptions of himself as a speaker should be congruent with his speaking behavior. It follows therefore that if a stutterer is fortunate enough to achieve speech that is free of stuttering, he should also perceive himself as a speaker who once stuttered or once was called a stutterer but is now a relatively fluent speaker.

The system of contingency management tends to divest itself of superfluous activity by the clinician. The clinician does what the program calls for. The clinician emits those behaviors that are designed to affect certain specified behaviors of the stutterer. He becomes specific, direct, and goal-oriented. Also, because the system is descriptive and process-oriented rather than just outcome-oriented, we are learning more about effective and ineffective clinician behavior.

The initial laboratory and clinical focus on developing tactics for establishing a new and stutter-free speech response has revealed the possibility of several effective procedures for this phase of therapy. We now see that changing the stutterer's speech pattern does not necessarily have to be a difficult or prolonged stage of therapy. As a result, a new emphasis is developing—one that is long overdue—on systematizing and programming the carryover phase of therapy. In this regard, greater attention is being given to the technology that is emerging in the self-regulatory therapies and to the principles of self-reinforcement.

Finally, some of the work emerging from the operant areas has implications for the prevention of stuttering. The work on parent-child interactions does not have to wait for the appearance of stuttering behavior to be applied to family systems. There may be implications in these projects for prevention in childhood of problems that go far beyond those of speech problems. The work on contingently suppressing stuttering through punishment and highlighting also has implications for prevention. The laboratory demonstrations of how these suppressive effects can be reversed are significant. By pairing punishment with positive reinforcement (Halvorson, 1971) and by preceding contingent punishment with random aversive stimulation of the same form (Brookshire, 1969; Brookshire and Eveslage, 1969) we see a partial explanation of the traditional view that punishment of dysfluency generates stuttering. These laboratory demonstrations that reversed the suppressive effects of punishment may be analogues of the stutterer's home situation, during which the use of punishment appears to be related to an increase in dysfluency. These studies possibly reflect that the traditional view of the role of punishment in the development of stuttering focused only on one aspect of the total paradigm—the use of punishment. Given such a narrow focus, it is understandable that we should have the traditional prescription that if you do not punish dysfluency or call attention to it, you can prevent stuttering. But it does not appear to be the punishment, per se, that generates stuttering. It is the way it is applied that could be detrimental. Contingent, suppressive stimulation could eventually become a preventative procedure, if the appropriately controlled tactics could be developed for its use in the home. If punishment is to be a useful preventative of stuttering, we would have to assure its consistent, contingent application and also prevent it from being paired with a positive, rewarding event. At this point, however, the complicated interactions of the family may defy such close control and contraindicate its use.

Much of this work is in its very early exploratory stages. It has been promising. However, we see too much fragmentation of effort. Individual enthusiasms fostered by successful laboratory and clinical demonstrations of operant approaches can insulate us from one another. Isolated projects must become integrated into programmatic endeavors whereby cooperative and collaborative action is systematically arranged. Although the end of the stuttering problem is not yet at hand, it is at least being hypothesized and conceptualized. To borrow and paraphrase a statement by one of the early pioneers in the field of stuttering, Robert West, the stutterer has done far more for us than we have ever done for him. Perhaps we are gradually reaching that point where we may be beginning to balance the scales and we are at least doing as much for him.

Bibliography

ABBOTT, J. A. Repressed hostility as a factor in adult stuttering. *J. Speech and Hearing Disorders,* 12 (1947) : 428–30.

ANDREWS, G. Editorial: Token reinforcement systems. *Australian and New Zealand J. Psychiatry,* 5 (1971) : 135–36.

———, and INGHAM, R. J. Stuttering: Considerations in the evaluation of treatment. *British J. Disorders of Communication,* 6 (1971) : 129–38.

BANDURA, A., and PERLOFF, B. Relative efficacy of self-monitored and externally imposed reinforcement systems. *J. Personality and Social Psychology,* 7 (1967) : 111–16.

BELLACK, A., ROZENSKY, R., and SCHWARTZ, J. Self-monitoring as an adjunct to a behavioral weight reduction program. Paper presented at APA Convention, 1973.

BELLACK, A. S. and TILLMAN, W. Effects of tasks and experimenter feedback on the self-reinforcement behavior of internals and externals. *J. Consulting and Clinical Psychology,* 42 (1974) : 330–36.

BERNE, E. *Games people play.* New York: Grove Press, 1967.

BLANTON, S. In *Stuttering, significant theories and therapies,* ed. E. Hahn, pp. 1–5. Stanford, Calif.: Stanford Univ. Press, 1958.

BLIND, J. J., SHAMES, G. H., and EGOLF, D. B. The use of verbal punishment in an experimental program of therapy for adult stutterers. Paper presented at American Speech and Hearing Association Convention, Detroit, 1973.

173

BLIND, J., EGOLF, D., and SHAMES, G. Critical factors for the carryover of fluency in stutterers. Paper presented at American Speech and Hearing Association Convention, San Francisco, 1972.

BLOODSTEIN, O. Stuttering as an anticipatory struggle reaction. In *Stuttering: A symposium*, ed. J. Eisenson. New York: Harper & Row, 1958.

———. The development of stuttering: I. Changes in nine basic features. *J. Speech and Hearing Disorders*, 25 (1960) : 219–37.

———. *A handbook on stuttering*. Chicago, Ill.: National Society for Crippled Children and Adults, 1969.

BLUEMEL, C. S. Primary and secondary stammering. *Quarterly J. Speech*, 18 (1932) : 187–200.

BOLSTAD, O. D., and JOHNSON, S. M. Self-regulation in the modification of disruptive classroom behavior. *J. Applied Behavioral Analysis*, 5 (1972) : 443–54.

BOOME, E. J. In *Stuttering, significant theories and therapies*, ed. E. Hahn, pp. 10–13. Stanford, Calif.: Stanford Univ. Press, 1958.

BOOTZIN, R. R. Stimulus control treatment for insomnia. Paper presented at APA Convention, 1972.

BORING, E. G. When is human behavior predetermined? *Scientific Monthly*, 84 (1957) : 189–96.

BROOKSHIRE, R. H. Effects of random and response contingent noise upon disfluencies of normal speakers. *J. Speech and Hearing Research*, 12 (1969) : 126–34.

———, and EVESLAGE, R. Verbal punishment of disfluency following augmentation of random delivery of aversive stimuli. *J. Speech and Hearing Research*, 12 (1969) : 383–88.

———, and MARTIN, R. R. The differential effects of three verbal punishers on the disfluencies of normal speakers. *J. Speech and Hearing Research*, 10 (1967) : 496–505.

BRUTTEN, E. J., and SHOEMAKER, D. J. *The modification of stuttering*. Englewood Cliffs, N.J.: Prentice-Hall, 1967.

BRYNGELSON, B. In *Stuttering, significant theories and therapies*, ed. E. Hahn, pp. 14–23. Stanford, Calif.: Stanford Univ. Press, 1958.

CARRIER, J., SHAMES, G. H., and EGOLF, D. The design and application of an experimental therapy program for stutterers. Paper presented at American Speech and Hearing Association Convention, 1969.

COOPER, E. B., CADY, B. B., and ROBBINS, C. J. The effect of the verbal stimulus words wrong, right and true on the disfluency rates of stutterers and non stutterers. *J. Speech and Hearing Research*, 13 (1970) : 239–44.

CORIAT, I. In *Stuttering, significant theories and therapies*, ed. E. Hahn, pp. 28–30. Stanford, Calif.: Stanford Univ. Press, 1958.

CURLEE, R. F., and PERKINS, W. H. Conversational rate control therapy for stuttering. *J. Speech and Hearing Disorders*, 34 (1969) : 245–50.

DAMSTE, H. A behavioral analysis of a stuttering therapy. In *Conditioning in stuttering therapy, applications and limitations*. Memphis: Speech Foundation of America, 1970.

DAVIS, D. M. The relation of repetitions in the speech of young children to certain measures of language maturity and situational factors, part I. *J. Speech and Hearing Disorders,* 4 (1939) : 303–18.

———. The relation of repetitions in the speech of young children to certain measures of language maturity and situational factors, parts II and III. *J. Speech and Hearing Disorders,* 5 (1940) : 235–46.

EGLAND, G. Reference cited in C. Van Riper. *Speech correction: Principles and methods.* Englewood Cliffs, N.J.: Prentice-Hall, 1954.

EGOLF, D. B., SHAMES, G. H., and BLIND, J. J. The combined use of operant procedures and theoretical concepts in the treatment of an adult female stutterer. *J. Speech and Hearing Disorders,* 36 (1971) : 414–21.

———, SHAMES, G. H., JOHNSON, P. R., and KASPRISIN-BURRELLI, A. The use of parent-child interaction patterns in therapy for young stutterers. *J. Speech and Hearing Disorders,* 51 (1972) : 222–32.

———, SHAMES, G. H., and SELTZER, H. The effects of time-out on the fluency of stutterers in group therapy. *J. Communication Disorders,* 4 (1971) : 111–18.

EPSTEIN, L. H., and PETERSON, G. L. The control of undesired behavior by self-imposed contingencies. *Behavioral Therapy,* 4 (1973): 91–95.

ERNST, F. A. Self-recording and counter conditioning of a self-mutilative compulsion. *Behavior Therapy,* 4 (1973) : 144–46.

FERSTER, C. B., and SKINNER, B. F. *Schedules of reinforcement.* New York: Appleton-Century-Crofts, 1957.

FETZ, E. E., and SMITH, O. A. Operant conditioning of precentral cortical cell activity in awake monkeys. *Federation Proceedings of the Federation of American Societies for Experimental Biology,* 28 (1969) : 521.

FINLEY, W. W. Effect of feedback on the control of cardiac rate. *J. Psychology,* 77 (1971) : 43–54.

FLANAGAN, B., GOLDIAMOND, I., and AZRIN, N. H. Operant stuttering: The control of stuttering behavior through response contingent consequences. *J. Experimental Analysis of Behavior,* 1 (1958) : 173–77.

———. In-statement of stuttering in normally fluent individuals through operant procedures. *Science,* 130 (1959) : 979–81.

FRICK, J. A. An exploratory study of the effect of punishment (electric shock) upon stuttering. Ph.D. dissertation, State University of Iowa, 1951.

GINOTT, H. *Between parent and child.* New York: Avon, 1969.

GLAUBER, P. The psychoanalysis of stuttering. In *Stuttering: A symposium,* ed. J. Eisenson. New York: Harper & Row, 1958, pp. 71–120.

GOLDIAMOND, I. Self-control procedures in personal behavior problems. *Psychological Reports,* 17 (1965a) : 851–68.

———. Stuttering and fluency as manipulable operant response classes. In *Research in behavior modification,* ed. L. Krasner and L. P. Ullman, pp. 106–56. New York: Holt, Rinehart and Winston, 1965b.

GRAY, B. B., and ENGLAND, E. *Some effects of anxiety deconditioning upon stuttering behavior.* Final report, Project No. RD-2021-S, Social and Rehabilitation Service, Dept. of HEW, 1968.

GREENE, J. In *Stuttering, significant theories and therapies,* ed. E. Hahn, pp. 55–58. Stanford, Calif.: Stanford Univ. Press, 1958.

HALVORSON, J. The effects on stuttering frequency of pairing punishment (response cost) with reinforcement. *J. Speech and Hearing Research,* 14 (1971) : 356–64.

HAROLDSON, S. K., MARTIN, R., and STARR, C. Time-out as a punishment for stuttering. *J. Speech and Hearing Research,* 11 (1968) : 560–66.

HOMME, L. E. Perspectives in psychology: XXIV. Control of coverants, the operants of the mind. *Psychological Record,* 15 (1965) : 501–11.

HONEYGOSKY, R. The conditioning of verbal expressions of anger. Unpublished research project, University of Pittsburgh, 1966.

INGHAM, R. J., and ANDREWS, G. Stuttering: The quality of fluency after treatment. *J. Communication Disorders,* 4 (1971) : 279–88.

———. Behavior therapy in stuttering: A review. *J. Speech and Hearing Disorders,* 38 (1973): 405–41.

INGHAM, R. J., and WINKLER, R. A comparison of the effectiveness of four treatment techniques. *J. Communication Disorders,* 5 (1972) : 91–117.

JOHNSON, C. Verbal conditioning of a stutterer in a therapeutic context. Master's thesis, University of Pittsburgh, 1966.

JOHNSON, W. In *Stuttering, significant theories and therapies,* ed. E. Hahn, pp. 59–70. Stanford, Calif.: Stanford Univ. Press, 1958.

———. Stuttering, treatment of the young stutterer in the school. *Speech Foundation of America,* 1964, p. 15.

KANFER, F. Self-regulation: Research, issues and speculations. Paper presented at the 9th Annual Institute for Research in Clinical Psychology, Behavioral Modification in Clinical Psychology, University of Kansas, 1967.

———. Maintenance of behavior by self-generated stimuli and reinforcement. Paper presented at the Conference on the Psychology of Private Events, Morgantown, W. Va., 1970a.

———. Self-monitoring: Methodological limitations and clinical applications. *J. Consulting and Clinical Psychology,* 35 (1970b) : 148–52.

———, and KAROLY, P. Self-control: A behavioristic excursion into the lion's den. *Behavior Therapy,* 3 (1972) : 398–416.

———, and MARSTON, A. Conditioning of self-reinforcing responses: An analogue to self-confidence training. *Psychological Reports,* 13 (1963) : 63–70.

———, and PHILLIPS, J. Behavior therapy: A panacea for all ills or a passing fancy? *Archives of General Psychiatry,* 15 (1966) : 114–28.

KASPRISIN-BURRELLI, A., EGOLF, D. B., and SHAMES, G. H. A comparison of parental verbal behavior with stuttering and nonstuttering children. *J. Communication Disorders,* 5 (1972) : 335–46.

KATKIN, E. S., and MURRAY, E. N. Instrumental conditioning of autonomically mediated behavior: Theoretical and methodological issues. *Psychological Bulletin,* 70 (1968) : 52–68.

KIMMEL, H. D. Instrumental conditioning of autonomically mediated behavior. *Psychological Bulletin,* 67 (1967) : 337–45.

KIESLER, D. J. Some myths of psychotherapy research and the search for a paradigm. *Psychological Bulletin,* 65 (1966) : 110–36.

KODISH, M., and TUCCIARONE, M. Increasing the average fluency interval: An individualized operant conditioning therapy program. Unpublished research, University of Pittsburgh, 1973.

KOLB, D., WINTER, S., and BERLEW, D. Self-directed change: Two studies. *J. Applied Behavioral Science,* 4 (1968) : 453–71.

KROUT, M. H. Emotional factors in the etiology of stuttering. *J. of Abnormal Psychology,* 31 (1936) : 174–81.

LANYON, R. Behavior change in stuttering through systematic desensitization. *J. Speech and Hearing Disorders,* 34 (1969) : 253–59.

LEACH, E. Stuttering: Clinical application of response contingent procedures. In *Stuttering and the conditioning therapies,* ed. B. Gray and E. England, pp. 115–28. Monterey, Calif.: Monterey Institute for Speech and Hearing, 1969.

LEFCOURT, H. Internal vs external control of reinforcement: A review. *Psychological Bulletin,* 65 (1966) : 206–20.

LEITH, W. R., and UHLEMANN, M. R. The shaping group: Theory, organization and function. Scientific exhibit at American Speech and Hearing Association Convention, 1970a.

————. The shaping group approach to stuttering: A clinical investigation. Scientific exhibit at American Speech and Hearing Association Convention, 1970b.

————. The treatment of stuttering by the shaping group. Paper presented at American Speech and Hearing Association Convention, 1970c.

————. The shaping group approach to stuttering. *Comparative Group Studies,* 3 (1972) : 175–99.

LOCKE, S., CARTLEDGE, N., and KOEPPEL, J. Motivational effect of knowledge of results: A goal setting phenomenon? *Psychological Bulletin,* 70 (1968) : 474–85.

MAHONEY, M. J. Research issues in self-management. *Behavioral Therapy,* 3 (1972a) : 145–63.

————. Self-control strategies in weight loss. Paper presented at the 6th Annual Meeting of the Association for the Advancement of Behavior Therapy, New York, 1972b.

————, MOWRA, N. G. M., and WADE, T. C. The relative efficacy of self-reward, self-punishment and self-monitoring techniques for weight loss. *J. Consulting and Clinical Psychology,* 40 (1973) : 404–10.

MARSTON, A. Variables in extinction following acquisition with vicarious reinforcement. *J. Experimental Psychology,* 68 (1964) : 312–15.

MARSTON, A. Self-reinforcement: The relevance of a concept in analogue research to psychotherapy. *Psychotherapy: Theory, Research and Practice,* 2 (1965) : 1–5.

MARTIN, R. R. The experimental manipulation of stuttering behaviors. In *Operant procedures in remedial speech and language training,* ed. H. Sloane, Jr., and Barbara D. MacAulay. Boston: Houghton-Mifflin, 1968, pp. 325–47.

————, and INGHAM, R. J. Stuttering. In *The modification of language behavior,* ed. B. Lahey, pp. 91–139. Springfield, Ill.: Charles Thomas, 1973.

————, and SIEGEL, G. M. The effects of response contingent shock on stuttering. *J. Speech and Hearing Research,* 9 (1966a) : 340–52.

————, and SIEGEL, G. M. The effects of simultaneously punishing stuttering and rewarding fluency. *J. Speech and Hearing Research,* 9 (1966b) : 466–75.

————, and SIEGEL, G. M. The effects of a neutral stimulus (buzzer) on motor responses and disfluencies in normal speakers. *J. Speech and Hearing Research,* 12 (1969) : 179–84.

McCANN, E. A study of the consistency of dysfluencies in the speech of non stuttering males of pre-school age. Master's thesis, University of Pittsburgh, 1967.

McFALL, R. Effects of self-monitoring on normal smoking behavior. *J. Consulting and Clinical Psychology,* 35 (1970) : 135–42.

————, and HAMMEN, C. Motivation, structure and self-monitoring: Role of nonspecific factors in smoking reduction. *J. Consulting and Clinical Psychology,* 37 (1971) : 80–86.

MILLER, N. E. Learning of visceral and glandular responses. *Science,* 163 (1969) : 434–45.

————, and DiCARA, L. Instrumental learning of heart rate changes in curarized rats: Shaping and specificity to discrimination stimulus *J. Comparative and Physiological Psychology,* 63 (1967) : 12–19.

NOWLISS, D. P., and KAMIYA, J. Control of EEG alpha rhythm through auditory feedback and the associated mental activity. *Psychophysiology,* 6 (1970) : 476.

PERKINS, W. H. Speech pathology: An applied behavioral science. St. Louis, Mo.: C. V. Mosby, 1971.

————. Replacement of stuttering with normal speech: I. rationale. *J. Speech and Hearing Disorders,* 38 (1973a) : 283–94.

————. Replacement of stuttering with normal speech: II. clinical procedures. *J. Speech and Hearing Disorders,* 38 (1973b) : 295–303.

QUICK, E. Self-monitoring and the control of overeating. Ph.D. dissertation, University of Pittsburgh, 1973.

QUIST, R. W., and MARTIN, R. R. The effect of response contingent verbal punishment on stuttering. *J. Speech and Hearing Disorders,* 10 (1967) : 795–800.

REED, C. G., and LINGWALL, J. B. An investigation of the relationship between punishment, GSR's and stuttering. Paper presented at American Speech and Hearing Association Convention, 1973.

REHM, L., and MARSTON, A. R. Reduction of social anxiety through modification of self-reinforcement: An instigation therapy technique. *J. Consulting and Clinical Psychology,* 32 (1968) : 565–74.

REHM, L., and ROZENSKY, R. H. Multiple behavior therapy techniques with a homosexual client: A case study. Unpublished research, 1973.

RICKARD, H., and MUNDY, M. Direct manipulation of stuttering behavior: An experimental and clinical approach. In *Case studies in behavior modification,* ed. L. Ullmann and L. Krasner, pp. 268–74. New York: Holt, Rinehart and Winston, 1965.

ROGERS, C. *Counseling and psychotherapy.* Cambridge, Mass.: Houghton-Mifflin, 1942.

ROTTER, J. *Generalized expectancies for internal versus external control of reinforcement.* Psychological Monograph 609, vol. 80, 1966.

ROZENSKY, R. H. The manipulation of temporal placement of self-monitoring: A case study of smoking reduction. Unpublished paper, 1973.

————. The tendency to self-reinforce as a diagnostic and predictor variable for success in self- versus externally controlled therapeutic programs for weight reduction. Ph.D. dissertation, University of Pittsburgh, 1974.

RUBIN, H., and CULATTA, R. Point of view about fluency. *J. American Speech and Hearing Association,* 13 (1971) : 380–87.

RYAN, B. An illustration for operant conditioning in stuttering therapy, applications and limitations. Memphis: Speech Foundation of America, 1970.

————. Operant procedures applied to stuttering therapy for children. *J. Speech and Hearing Association,* 36 (1971) : 264–80.

————, and VAN KIRK, B. A. Programmed stuttering therapy for children. Paper presented at American Speech and Hearing Association Convention, 1973.

————, and VAN KIRK, B. The establishment, transfer and maintenance of fluent speech in 50 stutterers using delayed auditory feedback and operant procedures. *J. Speech and Hearing Disorders,* 39 (1974) : 3–10.

SCHWARTZ, G. E. Cardiac responses to self-induced thoughts. *Psychophysiology,* 6 (1970) : 650.

SHAMES, G. H. Dysfluency and stuttering. *Pediatric Clinics of North America,* 15 (1968) : 691–704.

————. Verbal reinforcement during therapy interviews with stutterers. In *Stuttering and the conditioning therapies,* ed. B. Gray and E. England, p. 99. Monterey, Calif.: Monterey Institute for Speech and Hearing, 1969.

————. Operant conditioning and therapy for stuttering. In *Conditioning in stuttering therapy,* ed. S. Ainsworth, pp. 17–35. Memphis: Speech Foundation of America, 1970.

————, and EGOLF, D. B. *Experimental therapy for school age children and their parents.* USOE, Final report, Project No. 482130, Grant No. OEG-0-8-080080-3525, Dept. of HEW, June, 1971.

————, EGOLF, D. B., and RHODES, R. C. Experimental programs in stuttering therapy. *J. Speech and Hearing Disorders,* 34 (1969) : 30–47

————, and SHERRICK, C. E., Jr. A discussion of nonfluency and stuttering as operant behavior. *J. Speech and Hearing Disorders,* 28 (1963) : 3–18.

SHAPIRO, D., and CRIDER, A. Operant electrodermal conditioning under multiple schedules of reinforcement. *Psychophysiology,* 4 (1967) : 168–75.

————, TURSKY, B., and SCHWARTZ, G. E. Control of blood pressure in man by operant conditioning. *Circulation Research,* 27 (1970) : 127–32.

SHAW, C., and SHRUM, W. The effects of response-contingent reward on the connected speech of children who stutter. *J. Speech and Hearing Disorders,* 37 (1972) : 75–88.

SHEEHAN, J. Conflict theory in stuttering. In *Stuttering: A symposium,* ed. J. Eisenson, pp. 123–66. New York: Harper & Row, 1958a.

————. In *Stuttering, significant theories and therapies,* ed. E. Hahn, pp. 110–22. Stanford Calif.: Stanford Univ. Press, 1958b.

SIEGEL, G. M. Punishment, stuttering, and disfluency. *J. Speech and Hearing Research,* 13 (1970) : 677–714.

————, and MARTIN, R. R. Experimental modification of disfluency in normal speakers. *J. Speech and Hearing Research,* 8 (1965a) : 235–44.

————, and MARTIN, R. R. Verbal punishment of disfluencies in normal speakers. *J. Speech and Hearing Research,* 8 (1965b) : 245–51.

————, and MARTIN, R. R. Punishment of disfluencies in normal speakers. *J. Speech and Hearing Research,* 9 (1966) : 208–18.

————, and MARTIN, R. R. Verbal punishment of disfluencies during spontaneous speech. *Language and Speech,* 10 (1967) : 244–51.

————, and MARTIN, R. R. The effects of verbal stimuli on disfluencies during spontaneous speech. *J. Speech and Hearing Research,* 11 (1968) : 358–64.

SKINNER, B. F. *Science and human behavior.* New York: Macmillan, 1953.

————. *Verbal behavior.* Englewood Cliffs, N.J.: Prentice-Hall, 1957.

SOBELL, L. C., and SOBELL, M. B. A self-feedback technique to monitor drinking behavior in alcoholics. *Behavior Research and Therapy,* 11 (1973) : 237–38.

SWIFT, W. B. In *Stuttering, significant theories and therapies,* ed. E. Hahn, pp. 130–34. Stanford, Calif.: Stanford Univ. Press, 1958.

TASTO, D. L., and HINKLE, J. E. Muscle relaxation treatment for tension headaches. *Behavioral Research and Therapy,* 11 (1973): 347–50.

THORNDIKE, E. An experimental study of rewards. *Teachers College J.,* Contributions to Education series, Monograph No. 580 (1933) , pp. 1–72.

TRAVIS, L. E. The unspeakable feelings of people with special reference to stuttering. In *Handbook of speech pathology,* ed. L. Travis, pp. 916–46. New York: Appleton-Century-Crofts, 1957.

TREON, M., TAMAYO, F., and STANDLEY, S. M. The use of GSR biofeedback in the modification of stuttering. Paper presented at ASHA Convention, 1972.

TROTTER, W. D., and BERGMANN, M. F. Stutterer's and nonstutterer's reactions to speech situations. *J. Speech and Hearing Disorders,* 22 (1957) : 40–45.

TURSKY, B., and SHAPIRO, D. Operant conditioning of systolic blood pressure. *Psychophysiology,* 5 (1969) : 563.

VAN RIPER, C. The effect of penalty upon frequency of stuttering spasms. *J. Genetic Psychology,* 50 (1937) : 193–95.

————. To the stutterer as he begins his speech therapy. *J. Speech and Hearing Disorders,* 14 (1949) : 303–06.

————. *Speech correction, principles and methods,* 3rd ed. Englewood Cliffs, N.J.: Prentice-Hall, 1954.

————. Symptomatic therapy for stuttering. In *Handbook of speech pathology,* ed. L. E. Travis, pp. 878–96. New York: Appleton-Century-Crofts, 1957.

————. In *Stuttering, significant theories and therapies,* ed. E. Hahn, pp. 139–43. Stanford, Calif.: Stanford Univ. Press, 1958.

————. *Speech correction, principles and methods,* 4th ed. Englewood Cliffs, N.J.: Prentice-Hall, 1963.

————. *The nature of stuttering.* Englewood Cliffs, N.J.: Prentice-Hall, 1971.

————. *The treatment of stuttering.* Englewood Cliffs, N.J.: Prentice-Hall, 1973.

WATSON, D. L., THARP, R. G., and KRISBERG, J. Case study in self-modification: Suppression of inflammatory scratching while awake and asleep. *J. Behavior Therapy and Experimental Psychiatry,* 3 (1972) : 213–15.

WEST, R. In *Stuttering, significant theories and therapies,* ed. E. Hahn, pp. 149–51. Stanford, Calif.: Stanford Univ. Press, 1958.

WILLIAMS, D. A point of view about stuttering. *J. Speech and Hearing Research,* 22 (1957) : 390–97.

WINITZ, H. Repetitions in the vocalizations and speech of children in the first two years of life. *J. Speech and Hearing Disorders,* Monograph Supplement, June, 1961.

WISCHNER, G. Stuttering behavior and learning: A preliminary theoretical formulation. *J. Speech and Hearing Disorders,* 15 (1950) : 324–25.

WITZEL, M. A., and SCHULMAN, E. The effect of a response-cost paradigm on the length of a stutterer's fluency interval. Unpublished research, University of Pittsburgh, 1973.

WOLPE, J. *Psychotherapy by reciprocal inhibition.* Stanford, Calif.: Stanford Univ. Press, 1958.

Index